Andrea A. Soerensen
Tokico M. Moriya

Occupational accidents in Mobile Pre-Hospital Care

Andrea A. Soerensen
Tokico M. Moriya

Occupational accidents in Mobile Pre-Hospital Care

Emphasis on Biological Risks

ScienciaScripts

Imprint

Cover image: www.ingimage.com

This book is a translation from the original published under ISBN 978-3-330-76206-0.

Publisher:
Sciencia Scripts
is a trademark of
Dodo Books Indian Ocean Ltd. and OmniScriptum S.R.L publishing group

120 High Road, East Finchley, London, N2 9ED, United Kingdom
Str. Armeneasca 28/1, office 1, Chisinau MD-2012, Republic of Moldova, Europe
Managing Directors: Ieva Konstantinova, Victoria Ursu
info@omniscriptum.com

Printed at: see last page
ISBN: 978-620-8-38297-1

SUMMARY

The aim of this research was to study occupational risks among professionals working in mobile prehospital care (APH), with an emphasis on accidents involving potentially contaminated material. The first aimed to identify accidental exposure to occupational risk factors among healthcare staff working in mobile APH, and the second aimed to analyse accidental exposure to potentially contaminated biological material (pbm) among healthcare staff working in mobile APH at a private mobile APH company in the interior of the state of São Paulo, which provides care both in urban areas and on highways. In the first stage, a descriptive documentary study was carried out using data obtained from 4,992 Roadside Assistance Files and notifications from the Specialised Services in Safety Engineering and Occupational Medicine - SEESMT. In the second stage, a descriptive, exploratory study was carried out using semi-structured interviews with 50 professionals from the mobile APH team, including firefighters, nurses, doctors, nursing technicians and ambulance drivers. The project was approved by the Research Ethics Committee. The data was analysed using Epi Info version 3.4.3. In the first stage, 54 exposures to occupational risks were detected, of which only six were notified to the SEESMT. Among the occupational risks, the risk of accidents stood out (64.8 per cent), followed by non-ergonomic situations (16.7 per cent) and biological risks (9.2 per cent). In the second stage of the research, from a sample of 50 professionals from the Pre-Hospital Care team, the majority (94.4%) were aged between 20 and 50; male (84%); had been working in the area for between six and 60 months (56%); and were vaccinated against HBV (92%). Of the professionals interviewed (56%) reported accidental exposure to potentially contaminated biological material, totalling 41 accidents. Of the accidental exposures to mbpc (70.7%) affected intact skin; (17.1%) percutaneous skin; (7.3%) mucous membranes; and (4.9%) damaged skin. The areas of the body most exposed to mbpc were the forearm (41.5 per cent), arm (21.9 per cent) and hand (21.9 per cent). The majority of accidental exposures to mbpc occurred when performing immobilisation procedures (39%), extrication (21.9%) and physical examination (19.9%). Blood was the most common biological material exposed (85%). As for the use of Personal Protective Equipment at the time of the accident, the majority were wearing denim overalls (95%), high boots (90.2%) and procedural gloves (63.4%). The most frequent post-accidental exposure behaviour was to seek medical advice (29.3%); serological tests were carried out (17.1%). The majority did not register the accident at work (78.1%). The most favourable situations for accidental exposure to mbpc were: emergency (46.4%); patient agitation (28.6%); rescue operations (25%); distraction (21.4%); stress (17.9%) and the presence of a large volume of potentially contaminated biological material (14.3%). The majority of those interviewed suggested measures to prevent accidents with mbpc. The results of the study, the interviewees' suggestions and the literature review subsidised general proposals applied to health professionals, and those specific to mobile APH, for the prevention and control of accidents involving MBPC.

Descriptors: Biosafety. Mobile pre-hospital care. Biological accidents.

SUMMARY

CHAPTER 1

INTRODUCTION

In Brazil, after the industrialisation and urbanisation of the population that began in the sixties of the last century, there was a significant increase in the number of victims of traffic accidents; this was a reflection of the large number of vehicles coming into circulation, the disorganisation of the traffic system, the general lack of supervision, the poor condition of the vehicles on the streets, the bad behaviour of drivers and the impunity of offenders (OLIVEIRA; SOUZA, 2003).

As a result of the increase in the number of people injured, there was a need for victims to be cared for outside the hospital environment, which in large urban centres was carried out by rescue and salvage groups from the Fire Brigade. As the population grew and the demand for victim transport services increased, specialised services had to be created.

Thus, in the last two decades of the twentieth century, mobile urgent and emergency Pre-Hospital Care (APH) began to be organised in Brazil; help is sought to reach the victim in the first few minutes after a health problem has occurred, requiring the provision of adequate assistance and immediate transport to a hospital that is properly hierarchised and integrated into the Unified Health System - SUS (WHITAKER, 1993; BRASIL, 2002).

In Brazil, the organisation of ambulance services for transferring patients between non-hospital and hospital urgent and emergency care units, whether public or private, is almost exclusively the responsibility of the Mobile Emergency Care Service (SAMU), the Fire Brigade and a few private companies (BRASIL, 2002).

Private companies have gained strength in the last two decades with the privatisation of state and federal highways. Most ambulance companies are located in large urban centres.

According to the state's comprehensive emergency care policy, priority for mobile APH services is to promote quality of life and health in the following areas: trauma, cardiovascular emergencies, gynaecological and obstetric emergencies, paediatric emergencies, psychiatric emergencies, metabolic emergencies and respiratory emergencies (Brasil, 2002). Therefore, mobile APH services must be operationally, technically and scientifically prepared to offer a quality and competent service, based on Ordinance GM/MS 2048 of 5 November 2002 (BRASIL, 2002).

The ambulances manufactured today are not comparable to those that existed in the 1980s, as they are better equipped and better suited to patient care; there are also specific training courses for mobile APH service teams. Even so, there is heterogeneity between the existing services.

Even the best companies working in mobile APH still face a number of problems that need to be overcome or minimised, such as lack of adequate team training; absence of specific protocols for infection prevention and control; lack of team safety when assisting victims in a hostile environment; difficulties for the team to access the victim; limited space to carry out procedures and manoeuvres both when the vehicle is stationary and when it is moving; professionals with a lack of technical and/or scientific qualifications and bio-psycho-emotional suitability to work in the APH; professionals with interpersonal relationship difficulties within the team; difficulties related to antisepsis processes for carrying out invasive procedures, handling potentially contaminated materials and equipment, disposing of waste resulting from care; disinfection of ambulances, among others.

It should also be remembered that trauma victims can present and carry a large amount of dirt inside ambulances, such as blood, secretions, excretions, bodily fluids in general, as well as dirt, asphalt and dangerous products such as various fuels, acidic, alkaline, oxidising and toxic agents. These dirt and products can increase the risk to the victim and also jeopardise the health or life of the rescue team.

The mobile APH team can be exposed to all kinds of occupational risks, i.e. physical (exposure to explosive agents, high temperatures, radiation, noise), chemical (contact with toxic products, handling medicines, disinfectants and others), accident (limited space and physical layout of the ambulance; inadequate lighting; assisting the victim while the ambulance is moving fast), biological (contact with microorganisms), and non-ergonomic (sudden, repetitive movements; uncomfortable, prolonged positions; excessive weight and stress).

Among the various problems mentioned, the author has been particularly concerned about the biological risks arising from exposure to potentially contaminated material (PCM).

Mobile APH team professionals experience emergency situations at scenes involving the handling of bodily fluids, such as large quantities of blood associated with the stress of the emergency situation, the condition of the victim, the location of the accident, the difficulty of accessing the victim and the actual assistance to be provided.

In view of the above and the scarcity of specific studies on accidental exposure to biological risks among mobile APH professionals, the question arises:

- What are the occupational risks experienced by the mobile APH team?

- What is the frequency of accidental exposure to biological risks among healthcare professionals working in mobile APH?

- What variables can influence the occurrence of accidents with potentially contaminated biological material among healthcare staff working in mobile APH?

Diagnosing a situation is fundamental for drawing up any health care programme (PEREIRA; MORIYA, 1994). It is believed that this study on accidental exposure to potentially contaminated material in mobile APH team professionals could, in addition to expanding knowledge on the subject, which is still scarce in the literature, contribute towards subsidising the planning and implementation of preventive and control measures for accidents of this nature.

CHAPTER 2

LITERATURE REVIEW

2.1 Mobile Pre-Hospital Care

Mobile APH can be defined as care that seeks to reach victims early after they have suffered an injury to their health (clinical, surgical, traumatic or psychiatric), with a risk of suffering, sequelae or death, thus requiring help and/or adequate transport to a health service, which can be carried out by services such as the Emergency Medical Assistance Service - SAMU, Rescue and private sector ambulances (FERNANDES, 2004; BRASIL, 2002).

In France, mobile APH has existed for centuries and began with the creation of the ambulance by the French doctor "Dominique Jean Larrey" (1766-1842), considered the "Father of Military Medicine" who, during the Napoleonic wars, named a light and fast vehicle the "flying ambulance", created to attend to the war wounded when they needed immediate care (HISTORY OF THE AMBULANCE..., 2006).

The word ambulance comes from the Latin ambulare which means to walk or move, a reference to the old medical care when patients were transported on stretchers or wheelchairs. Originally the word meant a mobile hospital that followed the movements of the army. The concept of an ambulance began in Europe at the time of the Crusades in the 11th century, with the Knights of St John who received instructions from Arab and Greek doctors on how to carry out first aid. These Knights then acted as emergency responders, treating wounded soldiers on both sides of the war on the battlefields and taking them to tents for more appropriate treatment (HISTORY OF THE AMBULANCE..., 2006).

For a long time, this segment saw little development and it was only after the two world wars (1914-1918 and 1939-1945) that greater emphasis was placed on the care of those wounded in combat, a fact that has become even more relevant in modern wars.

In Brazil, mobile APH originated in July 1986 with the Rio de Janeiro State Fire Department's Rescue and Emergency Group (GSE/CBERJ). The team consisted of a doctor trained in APH, a firefighter rescuer, a nursing technician and a driver trained in rescue and first aid (FIGUEIREDO, 1996).

According to Whitaker, Gutierrez and Koizumi (1998), in the municipality of São Paulo in 1990, emergency care was structured on a model based fundamentally on the disorganised removal of serious patients to public referral hospitals, which generated a backlog of patients in these services.

Following the Ministry of Health's 1990/95 Five-Year Health Plan, which provided for the structuring of emergency care systems, existing APH services were improved and others implemented (BRASIL, 1991).

A major impetus for the participation of health teams in mobile APH was the creation of the Emergency Medical Assistance Service (Serviço de Atendimento Médico de Urgência - SAMU) in the city of São Paulo in February 1990, through a resolution between the State Health Department and the São Paulo State Public Security Department, and later through the privatisation of federal and state highways (WHITAKER, 1993; FERREIRA, 1999b). This participation became so important that several resolutions were issued, culminating in the publication of Ordinance GM/MS No. 2048, of 5 November 2002, which regulates emergency services, including mobile services, with a specific topic for Highway Concessionaires (BRASIL, 2002).

According to the Ordinance op. cit, primary mobile prehospital care is that which is carried out when the request for an ambulance is made by a citizen; secondary prehospital care is that which is carried out when the request is made by a health service where the patient has already received the first care necessary to stabilise the emergency condition, but needs to be taken to another more complex service to continue treatment.

The term ambulance is defined, according to GM/MS Ordinance 2048/2002, "as a vehicle (land, air or water) intended exclusively for the transport of sick people"; they are classified into six types, using letters from the alphabet, from A to F, according to the complexity of the care and the equipment and materials required for each type of vehicle to maintain life.

Type A, Transport Ambulance, is intended for the transport of patients in the horizontal decubitus position, who are not life-threatening, for simple and elective removals; the crew must be made up of two professionals, one being the driver and one a nursing technician or assistant. Type B, Basic Support Ambulance, is intended for pre-hospital transport of patients with an unknown risk to life and for inter-hospital transport, containing only the minimum life-sustaining equipment; the crew must be made up of two professionals, one being the driver and one a nursing technician or assistant. Type C, Rescue Ambulance, is intended for pre-hospital emergency care of patients with unknown life-threatening conditions, containing the necessary life-sustaining equipment; the crew must be made up of three military professionals, road police officers, military firefighters, and/or other professionals trained and certified in rescue and basic support. Type D, Advanced Support Ambulance (ASA) or Mobile ICU Ambulance, is designed to transport high-risk patients in pre-hospital emergencies and inter-hospital transport and must have the necessary medical equipment for this function; the crew must be made up of three professionals, one of whom is the driver, a nurse and a doctor. Type E, Medical Transport Aircraft, fixed or rotary wing, is used to transport patients by air. It is equipped with medical equipment approved by the competent bodies. This type is often used to transport patients who are in a city that is difficult to access or critical patients who need emergency care and are far from the destination hospital; care provided by aircraft should always be considered advanced life support, and for primary non-traumatic and secondary mobile pre-hospital care, the crew should be made up of the pilot, a doctor and a nurse. For traumatic emergencies and those requiring rescue, the presence of a trained professional is essential. Type F, Medical Transport Vessel, is a motorised waterway vehicle designed to transport patients by sea or river. All of them must have the necessary medical equipment to care for patients, depending on their severity.

The mobile APH team should be made up of two or three professionals depending on the type of care to be carried out; it must always include the driver of the boat and a nursing assistant/technician in cases of basic life support, as well as a doctor and a nurse in cases of advanced life support (BRASIL, 2002).

NBR 14561/2000 sets out the standards that must be met with regard to the dimensions and other specifications of the land vehicle (ABNT, 2000).

Mobile APH services must be staffed by a multi-professional team, both health professionals and non-health professionals, given that emergencies are not a medical or nursing speciality. The health professionals who make up the mobile APH team are: a doctor, a nurse, a nursing technician and a nursing assistant, both of whom work under the immediate supervision of the nurse. Other professionals should include: telephone operators, radio operators, emergency vehicle drivers, security professionals (military police, road police or other professionals) and military firefighters (BRASIL, 2002).

Ordinance GM/MS 2048/2002 describes the general requirements for the position and the competences/attributions of each worker (BRASIL, 2002).

The motorway concession notice states that one of the delegated services should be the specific provision of support to users, including, among other things, first aid and medical care for victims of traffic accidents, with possible removal to hospitals (SÃO PAULO, 1998).

With motorway concessionaires, from 1998 onwards, the mobile APH service on motorways was set up to provide urgent and emergency care to all users travelling on privatised motorways.

The Federal Council of Medicine (CFM), in its Resolution 1451/95, defines urgency as "the unforeseen occurrence of a health problem with or without potential risk to life, the sufferer of which requires immediate medical assistance" and emergency as "the medical confirmation of health problems that imply an imminent risk to life or intense suffering, thus requiring immediate medical treatment" (BRASIL, 1995).

The mobile APH that provides assistance to victims in clinical or traumatic urgencies and emergencies in urban areas predominantly attends to emergencies such as strokes, acute myocardial infarctions (AMI), among others. It also provides assistance in chaotic and highly dangerous situations, such as fires, assaults involving Firearm Injuries (FAF) or White Weapon Injuries (FAB), in a hostile urban environment; while in mobile APH, which provides assistance to victims in clinical or traumatic urgency and emergency situations on motorways, the teams work in accidents with multiple victims, entrapment in roadworks, scenes that may involve large quantities of organic fluids, especially blood, toxic products and/or explosives.

> The growth of companies operating in mobile APH has provided professionals with the opportunity to

However, many of them still have insufficient knowledge to be able to work properly, given that their technical or undergraduate courses offer, when they do, little specific theoretical and practical knowledge, which has a negative impact on their ability to work and develop in APH.

Thus, it is of fundamental importance that professionals who come to work in mobile APH should be qualified by the Emergency Education Centres, whose creation is indicated in the Regulation contained in Ordinance GM/MS 2048/2002, and fulfil the minimum curricular content proposed in the regulation.

2.2 Occupational risks

In common sense, risk can be defined as the possibility of the occurrence of a fact or event that brings danger; it is the fear or apprehension of anything that could cause us harm or harm (FERREIRA, 1999a).

Deslandes et al. (2002) define risk in terms of the logic of the game, stating that risk is the probability of an event occurring, combined with the magnitude of the losses and gains that this may entail.

Recently, the concept of risk has been strongly associated with negative results. This connotation creates a problematic field for the notion of "taking risks", excluding any recognition of (real or perceived) benefits. In this way, occupational risks stem from the rupture of a relationship between the worker and the work and production processes, and come from the probability of a certain event occurring (SÊCCO et al., 2005).

According to Galafasi (1999), occupational risks are all the conditions that can cause damage to workers' health in the workplace.

Burgues (1997) considers risks to workers' health to be all environmental factors that have the potential to cause injury, illness, disability or affect their well-being and that of the community.

According to Bulhões (1998), occupational risks in the workplace can be real, hidden or latent. Risks can be hidden due to lack of knowledge, information or ignorance, in which case the worker does not suspect their existence. Among the reasons that contribute to risks being hidden are irresponsibility, incompetence and profit over personal safety. Latent risk manifests itself in emergency and stress situations; workers know they are exposed to risk, but working conditions force them to expose themselves to it. Real risk is risk that is known to everyone, but cannot be solved or controlled due to the lack of solutions, high costs or lack of political will.

Ministry of Labour and Employment (MTE) Ordinance No 485 of 11 November 2005 (BRASIL, 2005b), published in the official gazette on 16 November 2005, provides for the implementation of measures to protect the health and safety of health service workers, as well as those who carry out health promotion and care activities in general.

In this Ordinance, in its Regulatory Standard (NR) 32, occupational risks are classified as physical, chemical and biological. Physical risks are the probability of exposure to physical agents represented by noise, vibrations, extreme temperatures, abnormal pressures, humidity, lighting and ionising radiation. Chemical risks represent the likelihood of exposure to chemical agents, represented by substances, compounds or chemical products in their various forms such as: dust, fumes, mists, fogs, gases, vapours, medicines, serums, among others. Biological risks are the probability of occupational exposure to biological agents, represented by microorganisms, whether genetically modified or not, cell cultures, parasites, fungi, viruses, protozoa, toxins and prions. The Ordinance also highlights actions related to the prevention of sharps accidents and the immunisation of workers.

Ordinance 485/2005 makes no mention of ergonomic and accident risks, which are mentioned in Ordinance° 3.214/78, which classifies occupational risks into five groups of risks: physical, chemical, biological, ergonomic and accident (BRASIL, 1994a). According to the 1978 Ordinance, ergonomic risk refers to all factors that may interfere with an individual's psychophysiological characteristics, leading to discomfort or health problems. These risks are represented by intense physical effort, manual lifting and carrying of weights, inadequate posture, rigid control of productivity, imposition of excessive rhythms, prolonged working hours, monotony, repetitive actions or other situations that cause physical and psychological stress.

In this study, we propose and use the term Non-Ergonomic Risk to represent all the factors that may interfere with an individual's psycho-physiological characteristics, leading to discomfort or aggravation of their health, resulting from intense physical effort, manual lifting and carrying of weights, inadequate posture, rigid control of productivity, imposition of excessive rhythms, long working hours, monotony, repetitive actions or other situations that cause physical and psychological stress. This change in terminology is due to the belief that ergonomic risk could not bring any kind of burden, since everything that is ergonomic is ideal for its use, preventing any kind of damage.

Accidental risks are those that put the worker in a dangerous situation, exposing their integrity and physical and moral well-being. They are represented by inadequate physical layout, unprotected machinery and equipment, inadequate or defective tools, inadequate lighting, electricity, the likelihood of fire or explosion, inadequate storage, the presence of venomous animals, or other risk situations that could contribute to the occurrence of accidents.

Mobile APH workers, like any other workers, are exposed to all kinds of occupational risks.

Identifying occupational risks is extremely important, as it allows us to control the causes of accidents of any kind, whether due to physical, chemical or biological agents that cause injuries, physical exertion and mental overload (ZOBOLI, 2001).

For Montgnier (1995) and Bulhões (1998), the hospital environment is unhealthy due to the presence of a series of biological agents that cause infection and infectious diseases in patients, healthcare staff and other hospital workers; situations that favour contact with blood and other bodily fluids; as well as insufficient or lack of material to work safely; among others.

It can be said that the mobile APH environment is as unhealthy as or even more unhealthy than the hospital environment, even when compared to higher risk sectors, due to the peculiar characteristics of the work carried out by the mobile APH team, associated with the location where the care is provided.

2.3 Biological risks and mobile APH

Every professional practice exposes its workers to some degree of occupational risk. Health professionals are no exception to this rule; the very nature of their work exposes them to a wide variety of occupational risks, especially biological ones. Some of the reasons for this include: the length of time workers spend in the hospital environment, which is considered unhealthy by nature due to the presence of various types of microorganisms, carrying out invasive or non-invasive procedures that expose workers to blood, secretions, excretions and other fluids, and potentially contaminated materials.

A wide variety of infectious agents can be transmitted during accidental exposure. In a review of the literature, Tarântola, Arbiteboul and Rachine (2006) described 60 different types of pathogens or species whose cases of transmission following occupational exposure in humans have been documented: 26 viruses, 18 bacteria/rickettsiae, 13 parasites and three yeasts.

According to MENDES (2003) the recognised routes of penetration of these microorganisms include: ingestion; inhalation through the upper respiratory tract; active or passive penetration through the mucous membranes; active or passive penetration through a solution of skin continuity; deposition on the skin followed by localised spread; introduction into the body through objects and instruments applied to muscle tissue or the bloodstream; by insect bites or animal bites.

Rodrigues et al. (1995) cite the existence of risks arising from improper handling of secretions, excretions, clothing, contaminated fields, sharps, rubbish and waste resulting from the execution of procedures, all carried out without standard precautions.

Accidental exposure to biological risks can lead to serious health problems and even death, the most worrying of which are those involving exposure to HBV, HCV and HIV.

Biological occupational risk for health workers has been a much-discussed topic in recent decades due to the serious problems it causes, not only for the individual exposed to the risk, but also for the family, the community and the state.

Until the emergence of AIDS, little importance was attached to accidents involving biological material; the focus shifted with the discovery of HIV, the causative agent of the much-feared AIDS, which is transmitted through contact with blood, secretions, excretions and other bodily fluids. In association with HIV, other viruses were included among the concerns of health professionals, mainly HBV and HCV.

There are several documented cases of accidental transmission, involving healthcare workers and patients, with hepatitis B and C viruses and human immunodeficiency virus - HIV (CDC, 2003; SANTOS; MONTEIRO; RUIZ, 2002, TEIXEIRA; VALLE, 1996).

According to Rapparini and Cardo (2004), even if they don't provide direct patient care, healthcare workers who work in healthcare units of any size, whether large, medium or small, are subject to a greater risk of acquiring infectious diseases through occupational exposure. Although the occupational risks of exposure to infectious agents are widely distributed in a healthcare institution, workers who come into direct contact with patients, mainly involving blood, secretions and other bodily fluids, are proportionally more vulnerable (APECIH, 1998).

For an infection to occur, three essential conditions are needed: an infectious agent with the capacity to infect and in sufficient numbers to produce the disease, a gateway for the agent to enter the guest, and a susceptible host. In addition to these conditions, other factors play a role in workers acquiring infections, such as the sector in which they work, the nature and frequency of exposure to the infectious agent, the activities they carry out, among others (GERBERDING, 1995).

Health professionals in the emergency services can be exposed to their patients' bodily fluids due to the unpredictable nature of their work (SPEERS, 2003),

In addition, working in mobile APH provides professionals with favourable conditions for accidental exposure to biological risks, due to: the peculiarities of the ambulance (limited, enclosed space, poor ventilation, recirculation of air, dynamics of traffic movements such as jolts, propulsion of the body by kinetic energies arising from accelerations or decelerations, sharp bends at high speed, among others); and the type of care (which involves stress arising from the very urgent/emergency situation of the condition, the need for invasive processes to maintain life, among others).

These exposures can be by direct contact with blood, secretions, excretions, other bodily fluids and infected lesions; or by indirect contact through splashes of blood, secretions, excretions, other bodily fluids from clients on the skin and/or mucous membranes; by transfer of pathogens through contaminated materials and equipment, aerosols and fomites.

We can't rule out the possibility of the opposite happening, i.e. the healthcare professional contaminating the patient directly, indirectly through the transfer of airborne pathogens, through fomites, or even through contaminated materials and equipment during use, due to a lack of proper decontamination, including cleaning and decontamination of the ambulance.

The possibility of contracting an airborne disease in confined spaces as a means of transport is a reality that cannot be ignored, as Moya (2007) points out. In theory, all respiratory diseases can be transmitted to health professionals in the course of their work. These include tuberculosis, meningitis, parotitis and measles, among others.

Alves and Bissel (2008) state that the patient with an infectious agent transports opportunistic or pathogenic microorganisms into the ambulance through coughing, urine, vomit, excreta or other exudates during pre-hospital transport; the deposited microorganisms can use the surfaces of the ambulance as a vehicle until they are inhaled, ingested, touched or inoculated to a subsequent patient or other members of the healthcare team.

The majority of studies on occupational accidents involving biological materials involving health professionals have been carried out in health institutions, and this is worrying, not only because of the high accident rates, but also because of the distance between the daily practice of health professionals and the knowledge already produced on the subject, and the neglect itself (BALSAMO; BARRIENTOS; ROSSI, 2000; BALSAMO, 2002; BREVIDELLI; CIANCIARULLO, 2002; SANTOS; MONTEIRO; RUIZ, 2002; RUIZ, BARBOZA; SOLER, 2004; MUROFUSE; MARZIALE; GEMELLI, 2005; BALSAMO; FELLI, 2006).

The literature review shows a significant number of studies on the subject of mobile APH, but only a small number deal with aspects related to occupational accidents. Among them are those that deal with exposure to biological risks and/or occupational accidents in general (NITSCHKE; LOPES; BUENO, 2000; TAKEDA, 2002;

ZAPAROLLI; MARZIALE, 2006; TAKEDA; ROBAZZI, 2007; SOERENSEN et al., 2008); adherence to standard precautions/use of personal protective equipment - PPE (FLORÊNCIO et al., 2003; VIANA; LOPES, 2005; LOPES et al., 2008; MAFRA et al., 2008); stress in pre-hospital rescue teams (AGUIAR et al., 2000); pathogenic bacteria in ambulances (ALVES; BISSEL, 2008); sanitary evacuation under biosafety conditions (MOYA, 2007).

The study by Florêncio et al. (2003) focuses mainly on adherence to standard precautions and mentions the frequency of accidents at work involving biological material among the rescue team; another study on adherence to standard precautions by the mobile pre-hospital care team in Belo Horizonte, Minas Gerais, (LOPES et al., 2008) also mentions the incidence of accidents at work involving biological material among the pre-hospital care team.

Two articles, one by Speers (2003) and the other by Patrick (2004) deal with the risks of contamination of mobile APH professionals with blood and other body fluids, but make no mention of accidental exposure rates.

An important aspect is the recording of accidents in order to understand the magnitude of the problem, to draw up and implement prevention and control measures and to monitor the injured worker. Studies carried out with healthcare workers have shown a worrying rate of underreporting and the reasons given for underreporting were that the injury was considered minor, unimportant, and there was no knowledge of the need for the Communication of Accident at Work - CAT (NAPOLEÃO, 1999; CANINI et al., 2002; MARZIALE, 2003). This situation persists despite Ministerial Order No. 777 of 2004, which made it compulsory to notify workers of various health problems, including accidents involving biological material (BRASIL, 2004).

The CDC, in 1988, considering the exposure of health professionals to blood and other biological fluids during the course of their work, introduced the adoption of protective measures known as Universal Precautions (UP), which were reformulated and classified as Standard Precautions (SP) in 1996 (CDC, 1988; CDC, 1996).

In 2007, a new manual on isolation precautions to prevent the transmission of infectious agents in healthcare establishments was published, adding new recommendations and reinforcing existing ones (CDC, 2007).

The recommendations of this document for PPs are as follows:

- Hand washing should be carried out before and after contact with patients, and between two or more procedures carried out on the same patient, and is also recommended after removing gloves and contact with equipment;

- The use of gloves is recommended if there is contact with blood or other potentially infectious liquids and when handling mucous membranes and non-intact skin.

- Wearing an apron is recommended if the worker's skin or clothing is likely to come into contact with blood or potentially infectious fluids;

- The use of a mask, goggles or face shield is recommended if there is a possibility of splashes of blood or potentially infectious liquids reaching the face.

- Decontamination of surfaces is recommended if blood or potentially infectious liquids are present;

- Articles and equipment must be cleaned and disinfected or sterilised before being used on another patient; handle them with gloves and wash your hands after handling equipment;

- It is recommended to sanitise clothes to prevent the transfer of microorganisms to people and the environment, using suitable machinery;

- In order to prevent accidents with sharps, there must be education on the use and disposal of these materials. Re-sharpening is prohibited. Used needles should not be broken or handled. They should be disposed of in rigid, impermeable and puncture-resistant boxes. Disposal boxes must be placed in suitable, visible and easily accessible locations. These materials should be transported carefully to avoid accidents;

- When resuscitating patients, ambuums or other equipment that prevents contact with the oral mucosa and oral secretions should be used;

- Single rooms should be prioritised for patients who are at high risk of transmitting or acquiring infections;

- For respiratory hygiene, symptomatic patients should be instructed to cover their mouths and noses with a handkerchief when coughing and/or sneezing and to put them in an appropriate place, to observe correct hand hygiene for hands containing respiratory secretions, to wear surgical masks when possible and to keep a greater distance between units;

- For safe practices during injections, prepare parenteral medications in a clean place, using aseptic technique, sterile and disposable materials;

- The use of masks is recommended during procedures such as lumbar puncture, epidural anaesthesia, intrathecal therapy; some studies describe the possibility of contamination by oropharyngeal secretion during some of these procedures;

- All healthcare workers should be vaccinated against the hepatitis B virus.

The use of PPE is a legal requirement. The employer must provide the appropriate type for the employee's activity and approved by the Brazilian Ministry of Labour, train the worker, require its compulsory use, replace the PPE when necessary and take responsibility for its hygiene and maintenance, and report any irregularities to the Ministry of Labour. The employee is obliged to use it only for the purpose for which it is intended, to store it, keep it and report any alteration that makes it unfit for use to the employer (GALAFASSI, 1999).

Many occupational exposures to biological material can be prevented by using safe techniques such as: not re-capping needles, folding and disposing of used ones in proper containers; using protective barriers such as gloves, masks, glasses, among others, when in contact with blood and other body fluids, can prevent accidental exposures that reach the mucous membranes (CDC, 2003).

Adopting biosafety measures with the aim of controlling infection is a moral and legal necessity, which makes the reason for the work true, values the professional and the profession in the eyes of society (CANALLI, 2008).

The CDC (2003) recommends adopting the following measures after occupational exposure to biological material:

Local care. Injuries resulting from accidents with potentially contaminated biological material should be washed immediately afterwards with soap and water. Mucous membranes and skin should be washed with plenty of running water or 0.9% saline solution. Caustic substances should not be used, as they only increase the size of the injured area.

Notification. Immediately after the accident, report it to the manager or unit responsible for dealing with accidents so that action can be taken. The ideal is to provide care within the first two hours and no later than 72 hours after the accident; the benefit becomes less and less as the hours go by.

The injured worker must be guaranteed the right to privacy and confidentiality; medical secrecy; to receive pre- and post-test counselling from a trained professional; to have initial and follow-up serological tests for HIV and hepatitis B and C; to receive chemoprophylaxis with antiretrovirals (ARV) for HIV for 28 days and prophylaxis for hepatitis B, when indicated. The accident and the measures taken must be recorded in the medical records, and the accident must be notified to the National Social Security Institute (INSS) by means of the Communication of Accident at Work (CAT), if the professional is hired under the Consolidation of Labour Laws (CLT). If the professional is a statutory employee, a file must be opened and sent to the State Medical Expertise Department (DPME) to report the accident at work.

Notification of accidents at work and occupational diseases at work is mandatory, according to Ministry of Health Ordinance 777 of 2004. Workers will be guaranteed their rights with regard to the recognition of an occupational disease in the event of seroconversion if these measures are taken (BRASIL, 2004).

For the state of São Paulo alone, the accident must be notified on SINABIO (only accidents involving biological material) or on SINAN, the Notifiable Diseases Information System (SÃO PAULO, 2007).

As for the source patient, the Principle of Autonomy must be observed, and in order for serological tests to be carried out, their consent is required, in a document signed by them and by two witnesses, and compulsory HIV serology is forbidden, except under court order. The source patient must be given sufficient information about the test that will be offered to them, and secrecy and confidentiality must be guaranteed. The results of the initial serological tests, if positive, should always be confirmed before informing the source patient. If the first HIV test on the source patient is negative, suspend ARVs for the injured professional (SÃO PAULO, 2007).

2.4 Mobile prehospital care in the context of biological risks

Among the infections/diseases identified as the main biological risks for healthcare workers are: pulmonary tuberculosis, viral hepatitis, Human Immunodeficiency Virus (HIV) and cytomegalovirus; Occasionally, workers can also be affected by diseases such as rubella, meningitis, diphtheria, herpes simplex, herpes zoster, chickenpox, typhoid fever, gastroenteritis, parotitis, epidemic keratoconjunctivitis and other diseases caused by bacteria involved in hospital infections such as Staphylococcus aureus, Echericha coli, Salmonella, Streptococcus, Proteus (BULHÕES,

1998).

2.4.1 Human Immunodeficiency Virus - HIV infection

AIDS is the most serious form of a spectrum of diseases related to HIV infection. This virus causes slow degeneration of the immune system, leading to the development of opportunistic infections and malignancies (NETINA, 2003). HIV is a retrovirus that infects defence cells (lymphocytes, monocytes and macrophages), destroying them. It binds to receptors on the cell membrane of TCD4 lymphocytes, multiplying in these cells, which are destroyed and progressively cause immunodeficiency (NETINA, 2003).

HIV has been isolated in blood, cerebrospinal fluid, semen, vaginal secretions, breast milk, saliva, tears, pleural, synovial and amniotic fluids. Its transmission has only been proven in the case of blood, semen, vaginal secretions and breast milk (BRASIL, 1994a).

It is transmitted through exposure to blood and its derivatives, sexual contact without proper protection, vertical transmission and infected breast milk (NETINA, 2003).

HIV is very sensitive to the external environment; it is estimated that it can live for around an hour outside the human body. Physical agents (heat, for example) and chemical agents (bleach, glutaraldehyde, alcohol, hydrogen peroxide) can quickly inactivate them (BRASIL, 1994a).

The Ministry of Health standard (BRASIL, 1999) on AIDS transmission in the workplace lists the situations that can favour occupational HIV transmission: parental exposure (needle sticks or cuts) and contact of mucous membranes with blood or other bodily fluids; exposure of the skin to blood, even if apparently intact, for a prolonged period of time or in large quantities. This standard warns that some health professionals, during their working hours in emergency units, come into contact with secretions or blood without paying due attention to the rules of biosafety; it points out that heroic behaviour in emergency situations is not justified and that the correct conduct should be guided by rationality, even in situations of proven emergency, when speed on the part of the professional does not invalidate the correct rules of biosafety being obeyed.

According to the CDC (2003), the risk of acquiring HIV infection from accidental percutaneous exposure to contaminated blood is between 0.2% and 0.5%, on average 0.3%; after exposure to mucous membranes, the risk is 0.1% and on damaged skin less than 0.1%. There are no reported cases of HIV infection acquired after exposure of intact skin to a small amount of blood over a short period of time.

To date there is no vaccine available with proven efficacy; some studies show that ARV prophylaxis can reduce the risk of acquiring HIV in the event of accidental exposure to blood and other body fluids. The CDC (2003) recommends it only for exposures that actually pose a risk of contamination, in view of its side effects.

Gerberding (2003) and Brasil (2004b) recommend that chemoprophylaxis for accidents involving biological material from a source known to be HIV positive or unknown, should be started up to two hours after the accident to prevent the virus from reaching the regional ganglia, or up to a maximum of 72 hours, with reduced efficacy. Animal studies suggest that chemoprophylaxis, when started 24 to 48 hours after exposure, is not effective. In order to follow this guideline, care should be provided as close as possible to the place of origin of the accident, so it is necessary for each unit to have a care programme up and running in order to minimise the time between the moment of the accident and care.

The administration of Post-Exposure Chemoprophylaxis in Brazil was recommended by the São Paulo State Health Department and the Ministry of Health in 1999. This document was revised in 2005 and currently sets out the recommendations for antiretroviral therapy (BRASIL, 2005a; SÃO PAULO, 2007).

Each accident must be carefully assessed by the team in charge in terms of the biological material involved, the type of accident and the source individual's HIV status.

Chemoprophylaxis, when indicated, should last 28 days. If it is negative, repeat it after six and twelve weeks and six months after the occupational accident. The rapid test is not indicated for exposed professionals (BRASIL, 2005a).

In situations where the risk of transmission is lower, basic chemoprophylaxis (two antiretroviral drugs) is indicated, preferably the combination of zidovudine and lamivudine, if possible combined in the same formulation. In cases of greater risk, expanded chemoprophylaxis is indicated with the addition of a protease inhibitor (nelfinavir or indinavir associated with ritonavir as a pharmacological adjuvant). The use of nevirapine in occupational post-exposure prophylaxis regimens is not recommended; there have been reports of serious adverse reactions with the drug in this situation. In situations of exposure with a high risk of resistance to one or more antiretroviral drugs normally indicated for chemoprophylaxis, the possibility of using alternative regimens should be considered. Due to the high drop-out rate observed in some studies, monitoring toxicity and adherence to therapy is recommended, regardless of the regimen chosen. In the case of accidents from an unknown source or patients with unknown serology, chemoprophylaxis is not recommended in principle, except in epidemiological situations of greater risk (BRASIL, 2005a).

It is recommended that the exposed professional take a period of observation during the HIV observation period of at least six months after ARV prophylaxis.

The injured professional should be advised not to fail to attend medical appointments; to use or request the use of condoms in any type of sexual relationship (vaginal and/or anal and/or oral); not to donate blood or other organic material; not to breastfeed and not to share syringes and needles (BRASIL, 2005a).

2.4.2 Hepatitis B

Hepatitis B is a communicable disease caused by the HBV virus. It is transmitted through unprotected sexual intercourse (semen and vaginal secretions), transfusion of contaminated blood and blood products, accidents with contaminated sharps, contact with the individual's skin lesions in the acute phase, oral route (saliva), breastfeeding, contamination by blood or infected fluids on the mucosa (BASSO, 1999; BALDY, 1997; SANTOS, 2002; NETTINA, 2003).

Man is the only natural reservoir of the hepatitis B virus, so chronic carrier status is responsible for the spread of the disease. Unlike HIV, which is sensitive to the external environment, HBV survives for around seven days in dried blood at room temperature (SANTOS, 2002).

The incubation period of the disease is around 45 to 180 days and can evolve without acute manifestations in most cases. Around 90 to 95 per cent of people develop a spontaneous cure and 5 to 10 per cent of those infected become chronic carriers, transmitting the virus for several years or throughout their lives (CDC, 2003).

The chronic form is characterised by a continuous inflammatory process of the liver lasting more than six months, which can evolve into liver cirrhosis and portal hypertension with episodes of digestive haemorrhages that usually lead to death. Hepatitis B is seen as the main cause of cirrhosis and hepatocellular carcinoma (NETTINA, 2003).

The risk of contracting Hepatitis B through a needlestick accident with contaminated blood ranges from 6 to 30 per cent and a minimal amount of contaminated blood is capable of spreading the disease (BRASIL, 2005a).

The likelihood of infection with the hepatitis B virus is significantly high and can reach up to 40 per cent. Compared to other infectious diseases, the risk of acquiring Hepatitis B is 100 times greater than the risk of HIV seroconversion and 10 times greater than the risk of acquiring Hepatitis C (CDC, 2003; BRAGA, 2000).

Because of these characteristics, the use of the hepatitis B vaccine is recommended for all healthcare workers and is available nationwide. Ideally, workers should be vaccinated during the training period. After completing the vaccination programme, a test should be carried out after about two months to check that the vaccine has conferred immunity.

Medicines for chemoprophylaxis, hepatitis B vaccine and hepatitis B hyperimmune immunoglobulin must be made available by public or private employers. Private hospital units must have Post-Exposure Prophylaxis drugs and hepatitis B vaccines purchased at their expense.

After exposure to biological material, if the worker has not been vaccinated, the use of the vaccine associated or not with hyperimmune gamma globulin for hepatitis B is effective in preventing HBV infection (CDC, 2003).

In addition to immunisation against HBV, control of blood and blood-derived products, the use of PP, not sharing materials that pose a risk of parenteral contagion, care when handling sharp materials, and the adoption of sterilisation, disinfection and cleaning routines for equipment and materials are also considered control and prevention measures (BRAGA, 2000; SANTOS, 2002).

2.4.3 Hepatitis C

Hepatitis C is considered a global public health problem. More than 180 million people in the world are chronic HCV carriers, of which 2 million are in Brazil (CIORLIA; ZANETTA, 2007).

Hepatitis C is transmitted after contact with contaminated blood and its incubation period is six to seven weeks.

The risk factors for acquiring HCV include blood transfusion, injecting drug use, HCV-positive sexual partners, and sex with multiple partners without using condoms (BRASIL, 2005a). Exposures involving blood or any other biological material should be considered at risk for follow-up purposes (RAPPARINI; CARDO, 2004).

The estimated risk of HCV transmission after percutaneous exposures is 3 to 10 per cent, after exposure to contaminated blood on mucous membranes and damaged skin it is not yet estimated, and on intact skin the risk is unknown (CDC, 2003).

The symptoms of hepatitis C are similar to those of hepatitis B, but less severe. Around 50 per cent of carriers develop chronic liver disease and 20 per cent progress to cirrhosis.

There is no specific effective measure for reducing the risk of transmission after occupational exposure to HCV. Studies have shown no prophylactic benefit from the use of gamma globulin or post-exposure interferon. The only effective measure for eliminating the risk of HCV infection is by preventing the accident from occurring and using PPs (BASSO, 1999).

2.4.4 Tuberculosis

The etiological agent of tuberculosis is the bacillus Mycobacterium tuberculosis and its transmission is via the respiratory tract through droplets of saliva (Flugge droplets) expelled by coughing, talking or sneezing by bacilliferous patients. Transmission can also occur indirectly through aerosols (ROUQUAYROL; ALMEIDA FILHO, 1999).

The risk of acquiring tuberculosis among health professionals depends on various factors such as: the prevalence of the disease, the profile of the cases seen, the area of work, the occupational group, the length of time working in the health area and the control measures adopted by the health institutions (RESENDE, 2004).

According to Raparini and Cardo (2004), among airborne occupational infections, tuberculosis should be given special attention due to its high transmissibility.

he World Health Organisation (WHO) (2002) recognises the unprecedented increase in the HIV-related tuberculosis epidemic, which deserves special attention. However, the adoption of an evaluation and follow-up programme for workers has not been carried out, especially in countries with a high prevalence of the disease (RESENDE, 2004).

HIV/tuberculosis co-infection alters the clinical behaviour and natural history of both. When HIV carriers acquire tuberculosis, they suffer a significant drop in their TCD4 lymphocyte count and an increase in HIV replication. Early diagnosis and treatment are essential for controlling tuberculosis in co-infected patients; rifampicin is essential for treating tuberculosis, given its inclusion in the treatment regimen.

CHAPTER 3

OBJECTIVES

3.1 General

To analyse the occupational risks faced by professionals in the Mobile Pre-Hospital Care (Mobile APH) team.

3.2 Specific

Identify:

1. Accidental exposure to occupational risk factors (accidents, chemical, biological, physical and non-ergonomic situations) among healthcare professionals in mobile APH;
2. The frequency of accidental exposure to potentially contaminated biological material (mbpc) among health team workers in mobile APH (nurses, doctors, drivers/rescuers and nursing technicians or assistants);
3. Situations favouring accidental exposure to mbpc among healthcare workers in mobile APH;
4. The body area most affected by mbpc accidents;
5. Behaviour adopted by workers in the mobile APH team when faced with an accident involving a mbpc;
6. Mobile APH workers' knowledge of the company's standards for preventing and controlling accidents with mbpc, training and protocol for behaviour in the event of accidental exposure;
7. The knowledge of mobile APH team workers on how to clean the ambulance, disinfect materials, package and dispose of mbpc;
8. List suggestions from mobile APH professionals on actions to prevent and control mbpc accidents;

9. Propose strategies to prevent and control accidents involving mbpc in mobile APH.

CHAPTER 4

METHODOLOGY

4.1 Nature of Research

The research had two distinct phases and equally distinct methods, both with a quantitative analysis approach.

In the first phase, a descriptive documentary study was carried out to achieve the first objective; in the second phase, a descriptive, exploratory study was carried out using semi-structured interviews to achieve the other objectives of the study.

Documentary research makes use of materials that have received non-analytical treatment, analysing primary source documents.

Descriptive research aims to describe the characteristics of a given population or phenomenon, or to establish relationships between variables; exploratory research aims to provide greater familiarity with the problem and to improve ideas or discover intuitions. Usually, descriptive research, together with exploratory research, is concerned with practical action and generally takes the form of a survey (GIL, 2002).

Data on the company was obtained through an interview with the Operational Director of the company's mobile APH service, a trained doctor specialising in traffic medicine.

4.2 Study site

It was carried out at a private mobile APH company in the interior of the state of São Paulo, which provides care in urban areas and on motorways. At the time the data was collected, the service had 120 employees (doctors, nurses, nursing technicians, drivers, firefighters and administrative staff), sixteen ambulances and fifteen operational bases at strategic points along the motorways.

The choice of this company as the field of study is justified by its performance in both urban and motorway services, the fact that its staff includes health professionals and that it is an active and experienced company in the mobile APH sector.

The company provides services to a private hospital in the city, so it carries out inter-hospital and APH transport in the urban area and serves two motorway concessionaires in the region, which cover 759 km of roads. One of them has six operational bases and the other nine, both of which make their bases available at strategic points along the highway, with a view to optimising service.

The company's mobile APH service is divided into two different types, depending on where they operate: mobile APH in urban areas and mobile APH on motorways, given that the skills required, training, psychological and physical profile, ambulance characteristics, equipment, materials, relationships and risks are different. Those who work in urban areas provide services at the homes of the company's partners or in the areas they call, where urgent and emergency services are provided in accordance with the contract signed with certain companies or localities. The team must treat, stabilise and transport patients who need hospital care. Basic Support Ambulances (ASB) transport low-risk patients and Advanced Support Ambulances (ASA) attend to and transport high-risk or unknown-risk patients.

The service that performs APH on highways has been operating since 1998, when the Highway Concessions Programme began with the privatisation of several stretches of state highway. With the help of the Fire Brigade and various courses (practical, theoretical, simulation, and others), the company's workers were gradually trained to perform APH on motorways. This has brought the Fire Brigade's professionals closer to the company and consequently increased their knowledge of equipment for rescue operations, which has made it possible to develop ambulances suitable for this task.

At the time of data collection for this study, the service consisted of one Advanced

Support Ambulance (ASA), two Basic Support Ambulances (ASB) at the company's headquarters and one ASA in a neighbouring town, for mobile APH in urban areas. For mobile APH on motorways, there were three ASAs, eight ASBs and one Rescue Vehicle.

The distinction made in this study between mobile APH on motorways and mobile APH in urban areas was due to differences in the characteristics of the ambulances and the type of care provided. The former allows more than one victim to be transported simultaneously; it requires equipment such as extrication devices; fire extinguishers; PPE for firefighting, extrication and dealing with dangerous products; tarpaulins for caring for multiple victims; ropes; chairs; carabiners, as well as equipment, among other things, for rescues at height and with a greater quantity of medication. All of this requires a much larger space and a detailed study in the accommodation of all the items to optimise space and weight distribution in the ambulance, for the development of the health team's actions with the patient(s).

The majority, i.e. 75 (12) of the ambulances, are used for road services and 25% (4) in urban areas.

4.3 Population

In order to achieve the first specific objective of this study, the reference population was made up of the Roadside Assistance Files (FAR) and the files of the Specialised Service in Safety Engineering and Occupational Medicine (SEESMT).

In order to achieve the other specific objectives, the reference population was made up of workers who work directly in mobile APH in urban areas and on motorways: doctors, nurses, nursing technicians or assistants, drivers and/or first responders and firefighters.

4.4 Sample/Inclusion Criteria

In order to achieve the first objective of the research, all the company's FARs and SEESMT records for the five-year period (from October 2000 to October 2005) were analysed. The FAR contains a detailed record of each service carried out by APH, which, in the event of an accident at work, allows the type of occupational exposure experienced by the service team and the risk factors involved to be identified. The SEESMT registration form is filled in when an accident at work is reported.

In order to achieve the other objectives, the sample included workers from the mobile APH team who work in urban areas and on motorways and who met the following inclusion criteria:

- Work in services that use type B, C or D ambulances;
- Have worked in mobile APH services in the labour market for at least three years;
- Have worked in the mobile APH area for at least six consecutive months;
- Be on call at the time of the interview;
- Consent to take part in the study, after verbal and written clarification about the research.

4.5 Procedures

Prior authorisation was sought from the technical director of the mobile APH service to analyse the FAR and the SEESMT occupational accident record and analysis forms, as well as to carry out the interviews with the mobile APH professionals.

The FAR contains data on the ambulance's travelling time, the date and place of the event, the destination hospital, the type of accident/trauma that occurred, scene assessment, user identification, trauma mechanism, patient assessment, medical conduct and nursing care, drugs and materials used, the professional category of the team and care complications. The latter includes accidental exposure of the professional. All this data was entered into the MS-Excel 2000 programme.

The SEESMT Record Sheets analysed the items on accidents at work and exposure to biological materials.

The SEESMT forms relating to accidents with biological materials contain information such as the injured person's personal details, the place/company where the accident occurred, the job position and function, the date and time of the accident, the time between the accident and care, previous accidents, the use of Personal Protective Equipment (PPE) at the time of the accident, the type of exposure, the material used and the act carried out at the time of the accident, the source patient, the behaviour and follow-up of the injured person.

The data collection instrument was drawn up based on the relevant literature and the experience of the author and supervisor. A semi-structured interview was carried out with professionals from the mobile APH team using a script with open and closed questions.

The interview script underwent content validation by three experts in the field and in research methodology, in order to check that the objectives set for this study could be achieved. A pilot test was also carried out with professionals from the population itself. No adjustments were necessary, which allowed the data from the pilot study to be included in this study's sample.

Data collection was carried out by the researcher at the operational bases (urban and motorway). During the data collection period, there was only one occasion when the entire on-duty team was on call.

4.6 Data analyses

The data was stored in a database using the Excel 2000 spreadsheet and then analysed using the Epi info software, version 3.4.3. It was arranged in tables and analysed using descriptive statistics.

The answers to the open questions were categorised according to similarity of content and entered into the database; some were transcribed to support the discussion.

4.7 Ethical and legal aspects

In view of the involvement of human beings in the research, the project was submitted to and approved by the Research Ethics Committee of the "Centro Universitário Barão de Mauá".

The interviews were carried out individually with the workers, in the service itself, in a place that afforded privacy to both the interviewee and the interviewer.

Before answering the interview, these workers received verbal information about the purpose, objectives and procedures of the research. When they agreed, they signed an informed consent form.

CHAPTER 5

RESULTS AND DISCUSSION

The results are presented in two parts: the first refers to data on occupational risk factors in mobile APH on motorways, obtained from SEESMT and FAR forms; and the second refers to data on accidental exposure to potentially contaminated biological material (pbm) in health team workers in road and urban mobile APH, obtained through interviews with the health team involved in this APH.

Part I - Occupational risk factors in mobile prehospital care on motorways

A total of 9976 Roadside Assistance Forms (FAR) were analysed, and 4984 (50%) were excluded because they were incorrectly filled in or had incomplete data. The sample of this study comprised 4992 (50%) FARs in which 54 exposures to occupational risks were detected, six of which were notified to the SEESMT. During the period of this study, 2000 to 2005, 163 workers were involved in mobile APH on the motorways.

Notification of accidents at work is necessary and of fundamental importance in order to subsidise any work to prevent and control accidents. However, there is alarming underreporting, not to mention the FARs that had to be excluded because they were incorrectly filled in or had incomplete data. According to Robazzi et al. (2006), the reasons for underreporting accidents at work can be diverse, such as fear of losing one's job, fear of punishment and also the employer's lack of interest, because in the face of an accident the company shows its aggressiveness in the workplace.

Under-reporting can also be related to a lack of guidance, neglect on the part of the injured person or another professional, as the notification form for accidents at work can be filled in by any professional. With regard to lack of guidance, GM/MS Ordinance 2048 (BRAZIL, 2002), which considers that there is still insufficient attention given to this area in undergraduate courses, states that professionals who come to work in mobile APH services, whether or not they come from the health sector, should be trained by the Emergency Education Centres. It is well known that this requirement is not always met for mobile APH teams. As for neglect, many people trivialise the accident, as in the case of accidental exposure to mbpc, placing themselves as invulnerable to contamination by infectious agents, or because they believe it is inherent to the type of work they do.

Table 1 shows the distribution of accidental exposure to occupational risks (n=54) among workers in the mobile APH team operating on motorways, according to the risk classification defined by Ordinance° 3.214/78 (BRASIL, 1994a).

Table 1 - Distribution of accidental exposure to occupational risks (n = 54) among mobile prehospital care workers, according to risk classification, between 2000 and 2005. Ribeirão Preto, 2007

Occupational risks	*f*	%
Accidents	35	64,8
Non-ergonomic situations	09	16,7
Biological	05	9,3
Physical	03	5,6
Chemicals	02	3,7
Total	**54**	**100**

Among the occupational risk exposures among the professionals in the mobile APH team, the risk of accidents stood out (64.8%), followed by non-ergonomic situations (16.7%) and biological risk (9.2%). Physical and chemical risks occurred less frequently.

Table 2 shows the types of accidents faced by workers in terms of the risk of accidents.

Table 2 - Distribution of exposure to the risk of accidents (n= 35) among mobile prehospital care team workers, according to type of accident, between 2000 and 2005. Ribeirão Preto, 2007

Types of accidents	*f*	%
Car collision	10	28,6
Aggression by the victim, family members and users	05	14,3
Falls and slips during access/approach to the victim	04	11,4
Hit-and-run accidents	03	8,6
Objects thrown from the road onto the worker	03	8,6
Stings by venomous insects	03	8,6
Fall during departure from the Operational Base	02	5,7
Injuries caused by bodily friction/contact in Hardware	02	5,7
Accident en route	02	5,7
Injuries caused by bodily contact with the inside of the ambulance	01	2,9

Total	35	100

Of the 35 accidental exposures to the risk of an accident, the most frequent event was a car collision with 10 (28.6%) occurrences.

When Zapparoli and Marziale (2006) carried out a study to identify the occupational risk factors to which professionals working in basic and advanced life support units in emergencies are exposed, they interviewed the workers and found that 90 per cent reported car accidents as a risk factor, corroborating the data from the present study.

When analysing this type of event, it was found that accidents occurred in different situations:

- Ambulance collision: in a tunnel (1), with the wall on the side of the motorway (2), with another vehicle as a result of its involuntary movement when leaving the User Assistance Service (1); with a motorbike during emergency care (1); with a tow truck (1); with an inspection vehicle (1); with a lorry carrying a live load (chicken) and subsequent overturning of the lorry (1).

- Ambulance overturns after colliding with the side of the road (1).

- Ambulance overturned due to collision with rear of lorry while approaching accident scene (1).

As for the aggressions suffered by the workers, the situations were as follows:

- the aggression of alcoholic victims, family members and users against the professionals of the mobile APH team (1);

- accident involving a stolen vehicle with exchanges of fire between the victims and the military road police (1);

- assault without cause recorded (3).

Physical aggression was mentioned by 90 per cent of workers as an occupational risk factor in Basic and Advanced Life Support and Emergency Units (ZAPPAROLI; MARZIALE,

2006). We agree with the authors that violence is a worrying risk factor and deserves to be investigated in order to help prepare workers to deal with these situations, with a view to promoting greater safety at work.

The WHO (2002) conceptualises violence as the use of physical force or power, threatened or actual, against oneself, another person or against a group or community, which results in or is likely to result in injury, death or psychological harm, impaired development or deprivation.

Corbert, Grang and Thomas (1998), when studying APH workers' exposure to violence and abuse, found that many of them felt angry or irritated after this type of occurrence.

Several factors may be involved in the occurrence of assaults on the mobile APH team, including the stress caused by the emergency situation on both sides, users and the mobile APH team.

The situations that led to falls and slips during access and approach to the victim were:

- grass or wet soil (1);
- holes covered by the bush (1);
- product spilt in the accident (1);
- water channel (1).

The falls while leaving the base were due to the carpet (1) and the wet floor (1).

The people who were hit were professionals from the mobile APH team, who were securing the scene and signalling the road (3).

Although they are not part of the APH team, two users who were watching the accident on the motorway were run over. Although this is not classified as an occupational accident, it raises the need to work on preventing this type of accident. There is a need for a wide-ranging effort to warn and guide users not to remain at the scene of the accident, as this not only creates other risk situations but also jeopardises the performance of the health team.

As for objects thrown onto the road, there were also accidental exposures caused by a lorry wheel coming off (2), one hitting an inspection vehicle and the other hitting the ambulance, and a signalling cone being thrown off the road during lorry traffic, hitting the ambulance (1).

With regard to stings by venomous insects, these were caused by marimbondos and bees during care (3). The FAR for these accidents does not specify the type of bee. In Brazil, the majority of recorded cases of stings are caused by Africanised bees, which originate from the crossing of European and African bees and are currently found throughout the country (PREVENÇÃO DE ACIDENTES..., 2001).

Oliveira et al. (2000) believe that accidents caused by bee stings should be reported, as it is important to increase knowledge about the variety of clinical manifestations.

The FAR also recorded the presence of snakes and scorpions in the operational base, putting the mobile APH team workers at risk.

In relation to collisions with ironwork, bodily injuries were recorded during the extrication of the victim (2), one of which caused a laceration to the scalp and the other a minor blunt cut injury to the forearm, with damage to the PPE, i.e. a jacket that is highly resistant to high temperatures. In this case, the importance of wearing PPE is clear, as it protected the worker from more serious injuries.

As for bodily impacts against the inside of the ambulance, skin injuries such as abrasions and bruises caused by sharp changes in direction or acceleration were recorded. During transport or when moving the ambulance, professionals who are not wearing seat belts could be thrown against objects and/or patients. Another aspect to be observed is the accommodation and proper securing of equipment so that it is not thrown against staff or patients.

In 2005, NBR 15292 was approved, which refers to High Visibility Safety Clothing, with a view to increasing the safety of workers exposed to vehicle traffic (ABNT, 2005). This standard establishes the type and performance of materials to be used in the clothing of professionals who need high visibility and safety to carry out their activities. It specifies the minimum areas of use and suggests the positioning of materials in order to increase visibility and, consequently, worker safety. The standard establishes occupational visibility classes on a scale of 1 to 3 (visibility class 1, visibility class 2 and visibility class 3) according to the activities carried out and their occupational risks. Emergency and rescue personnel on public roads (medical teams, firefighters, and others) fall into visibility class 3, i.e. they must be highly visible, surpassing class 1 and 2.

Workers with class 3 visibility requirements must use combined performance retro-reflective material on their uniforms, which is capable of allowing retro-reflection of light in order to increase visibility in low or no light environments, or in adverse conditions such as rain, smoke or fog. The combined performance retro-reflective material also provides fluorescence, which is the property of emitting optical radiation of longer wavelengths than absorbed. This material increases daytime visibility, especially at dawn and dusk.

The material must also have some essential physical characteristics, such as being breathable, colourfast to cleaning and resistant to: rubbing, ironing, household cleaning, traction, abrasion, breaking, tearing, exposure to temperature variations, washing and being repellent to water penetration. The standard also includes design suggestions for garments such as trousers, long-sleeved shirts and jackets or long-sleeved overalls.

During the interviews with the workers, who were the subjects of the research, it was observed that they were not wearing uniforms as recommended by NBR 15292 (ABNT, 2005).

With regard to accidents on the road, the worker's motorbike fell (2), one on the urban road during the journey (company/residence) and the other on the motorway.

Among the occupational risk exposures, nine non-ergonomic situations were recorded, five of which were characterised by lumbar pain due to handling/moving the board while transporting the patient; one by a bruised wrist while lifting the board under an obese elderly patient; one by a dislocated knee while lifting the board; two by psychological stress due to a violent death resulting from a traffic accident on the motorway.

A study by Takeda and Robazzi (2007) of ambulance drivers showed that the highest frequency of accidents was due to excessive exercise and vigorous, repeated movements, characterising a non-ergonomic situation.

Emergency care requires the professional to act quickly and precisely, with a high level of cognitive and psychomotor skills (REIS; CORREA, 1990). However, it is important to emphasise that these actions are carried out in the most varied environments, ranging from the interior of an ambulance with limited space and in motion to the most unusual places, such as in the middle of hardware, toxic, explosive or slippery substances, hostile environments such as fires, landslides, scenes of violence, psychological pressure on the victim(s) and carers, among others. These situations require workers to lift weights to transport the victim(s) and equipment, use rescue equipment specific to the situation, repetitive movements, uncomfortable, inappropriate and prolonged postures, bending the spine, and others that can affect the worker's physical and mental health, often irreversibly.

The type of transport for a traumatised patient varies according to the situation, such as the presence of danger at the scene, the number of rescuers available, the diagnosis, the severity and the scene of the trauma; when not transported properly it can cause a second trauma and the rescuer can suffer muscle or spinal injuries, burns and electric shock, among others (FIGUEIREDO et al., 1997).

A large number of accidents, due to non-ergonomic situations, are perhaps under-reported due to workers trivialising their signs and symptoms (fatigue, low back pain, myalgia, anxiety, physical and mental exhaustion) because they believe them to be inherent to the very nature of mobile APH work.

The risk of a biological accident in this study was identified in 5 (9%) workers. The situations found were as follows:

- Oral contamination in sewage during water rescue, causing gastroenterocolitis (1);
- Exposure to vomit that hit the worker's face (1);
- Accidental exposure with mbpc-contaminated sharps that hit the hand (1);
- Exposure of damaged skin to blood (2).

Mobile APH assists clients with a variety of pathologies, including infectious ones, and victims of various types of trauma that can generate major bleeding, exceptions, secretions and other bodily fluids. A patient with an infectious agent can pass opportunistic or pathogenic microorganisms to the ambulance through coughing, urine, vomit, excreta or other exudates during pre-hospital transport. The deposited microorganisms can use the surfaces of the ambulance as fomites until they are inhaled, ingested, touched, inoculated to a subsequent patient, or even to other members of the healthcare team (ALVES; BISSEL, 2008).

Workers in this segment are faced with the most diverse and complicated situations peculiar to mobile pre-hospital care. The place of assistance can be in the environment where the victim(s) are: hostile environment, with poor lighting, danger of explosion, fire, rough and/or slippery terrain, pressure from family members and onlookers, among others; carrying out care in a wide variety of places with a high potential for biological risk, as in the case of sewage; or carrying out care in the ambulance with limited space under the action of the dynamics of traffic movements, such as shaking, propulsion of the body by the energies of traffic resulting from accelerations and decelerations, sharp bends at high speed, among others. It is important to emphasise that this type of care involves stress due to the very urgent/emergency nature of the situation and the need for invasive processes to maintain life. All of these factors provide staff with favourable conditions for accidental exposure to biological risks, either through direct contact with blood, secretions, excretions, other bodily fluids, and infected lesions; or through indirect contact via splashes of blood, secretions, excretions, other bodily fluids from clients, on the skin and/or mucous membranes; by transferring pathogens through contaminated materials and equipment, aerosols and fomites.

In the study carried out by Zapparoli and Marziale (2006), 100 per cent of the interviewees mentioned the possibility of acquiring an infection as a risk factor when working in medical care in basic and advanced life support units in emergencies. This demonstrates the perception of mobile APH workers regarding their vulnerability to accidental exposure to biological risks arising from their own experience in the field.

PPs came about to increase the safety of healthcare professionals when carrying out activities that expose them to blood, secretions, excretions and other bodily fluids.

Alves and Bissell (2008) agree that the PP and equipment available can reduce the biological risks to patients and providers, but the ambulance remains vulnerable to contamination by biological secretions.

According to Sarquis and Felli (2000), although there is the possibility of preventing accidental exposure to mbpc with the use of personal protective equipment (PPE), gloves, masks, aprons, caps and boots, with an emphasis on hand hygiene and care with sharps, the care taken with these precautions is not always practised.

In the study carried out by Mafra et al. (2008) on the importance of using PPE for biological risks in a mobile emergency care service, it was found that nurses are aware of the importance of using PPE, but do not use it frequently enough in their daily work.

In this study, two exposures to chemical risks were detected, specifically to sodium hypochlorite.

The situations that led the professionals on the mobile APH team to be accidentally exposed to the chemical risk was the use of sodium hypochlorite to clean and decontaminate the ambulance. An important detail reported by the interviewees is that the cleaning procedure was carried out on a very sunny and hot day, which favoured the inhalation of sodium hypochlorite fumes, causing exogenous intoxication.

Despite the multiplicity of chemical products that exist in the world of health work, the workers who handle them don't seem to be able to relate them to the chemical risk.

According to Takeda (2002), ambulance drivers regularly handle sodium hypochlorite when carrying out concurrent vehicle disinfection and are also subject to inhaling chemical agents from car combustion (carbon monoxide), which can damage their health.

According to Prista and Uva (2000), chemical risk factors are one of the most numerous groups of occupational disease agents.

The International Programme on Chemical Safety estimates that there are 100,000 pure chemical substances; 4 million compounds with commercial use; and several hundred synthetic chemicals introduced into the human living environment every year (PRISTA; UVA, 2000).

According to the WHO, of the 100,000 chemical substances considered to be agents of occupational illness, 200 to 300 are mutagenic and carcinogenic and more than 100,000 are allergenic and/or irritant (PRISTA; UVA, 2008).

Healthcare professionals are exposed to chemical risks generated by handling a wide variety of chemical substances and administering medicines, which can cause allergies, poisoning, irritation, mutations and even neoplasms.

In addition to handling and administering medicines, mobile APH workers can be exposed to various chemical products when dealing with accidents. The consequences of chemical exposure don't always appear immediately or in the short term, but can take months or even years, which is why it's difficult to report this type of accident.

The Pan American Health Organisation uses the terms chemical accident and chemical emergency:

> "a hazardous event or situation that results from the release of substances that pose a risk to human health and/or the environment in the short or long term. These events or situations include fires, explosions, leaks or releases of toxic substances that can cause illness, injury, disability or death to large numbers of people" (PANAMERICAN HEALTH ORGANISATION, SAO PAULO, 1998).

Because of the type of assistance they provide, mobile APH workers are exposed to a range of situations including fires, explosions, leaks or releases of toxic substances, and are therefore exposed to the risks of chemical accidents.

In a literature review on the chemical risks to which nursing workers are exposed, Xelegati and Robazzi (2003) identified in the publications found the main agents that can favour contact with these risks and cause health changes in nursing workers; they found fewer studies on chemical risks than on other risks; they warned of the need for more research on the subject, with the aim of increasing existing knowledge and facilitating awareness among the workers themselves.

As for physical risks (3), they mentioned bad weather (rain, cold, frost), which caused two cases of pneumonia and one upper airway infection (UAI).

Mobile APH workers are exposed to all kinds of physical risks: radiation, vibrations, noise, ambient temperature, lighting and electricity.

In short, the situations they experience are unpredictable and "can be exacerbated by the nature of the care provided, often in extremely complex situations, such as the kinematics of the trauma, difficult-to-access locations, the stress of handling care quickly and others" (MAFRA et al., 2008, p. 33).

Part II - Accidental exposure to potentially contaminated biological material (mbpc) in healthcare professionals in mobile APH

Of the 54 workers contacted, three had been working in mobile APH for less than six months and one was not interested in taking part in the study, so they were excluded. Fifty (41.6%) professionals from the mobile APH team at a private institution took part in the study through interviews.

Table 3 shows the characterisation of the mobile APH team according to age, gender, profession, length of professional training, time working in the mobile APH area, accidental exposure to mbpc, and vaccination against the hepatitis B virus.

Table 3 - Characterisation of mobile prehospital care staff (n=50) in terms of age, gender, profession, length of professional training, time working in the area, type of mobile APH, accidental exposure to potentially contaminated biological material and vaccination against the hepatitis B virus. Ribeirão Preto, 2007

Variables	*f*	%
Age group (years)		
20 |- 30	19	38,0
31 |- 40	12	24,0
41 |- 50	16	32,0
>51	03	6,0
Sex		
Male	42	84,0
Female	08	16,0
Profession		
Doctor	06	12,0
Nurse	08	16,0
Fireman	15	30,0
Nursing technician	12	24,0
Driver	09	18,0
Length of professional training (months)		
06 |- 60	13	26,0
61 |- 120	14	28,0
>121	23	46,0
Length of service (months)		
06 |- 60	28	56,0
61 |- 120	12	24,0
>121	10	20,0
Type APH		
APH on motorways	40	80,0
APH in urban areas	10	20,0
Accidental exposure to mbpc		
Yes	28	56,0
No	22	44,0

Vaccination against the hepatitis B virus		
Yes	46	92,0
No	04	8,0

As for the characterisation of the mobile APH team, the majority (94.4%) of those interviewed were aged between 20 and 50; were male (84.0%); were firefighters (30%); had more than 120 months' professional training (46%); had been working in the area for between six and 60 months (56%); worked in mobile APH on highways (80%); had been accidentally exposed to mbpc (56%) and had been vaccinated against HBV (92%).

Ordinance GM/MS No. 2048 of 2002 (BRASIL, 2002) states that the profile required of doctors, nurses, nursing technicians, nursing assistants and firefighters to work in APH is: emotional balance and self-control; willingness to carry out guided actions; physical and mental capacity for the activity, manual and physical dexterity to work in mobile units; availability for the training detailed in the ordinance in question, as well as for recertification, among others specific to each area of professional activity.

In addition to age, gender and length of professional training and experience in the field are factors that can contribute, in part, to greater or lesser suitability for the profile required to work in APH, which requires specific knowledge, as well as other attributes such as agility, strength, endurance and physical mobility.

In terms of job category, firefighters appear most frequently (30 per cent), followed by nursing technicians, drivers and, less frequently, nurses and doctors.

This multidisciplinary nature of the mobile APH team is important because it brings together different types of expertise and different types of activity. The firefighter can provide practical and theoretical knowledge about the whole process of rescue, extrication of victims, among other activities, knowledge that is more specific to this area and which nurses and doctors have little control over.

Only integrated action by all professionals, whether or not they come from the health sector, can result in adequate specialised care outside of hospital, aimed at maintaining life and/or minimising sequelae.

The number of each professional in the mobile APH team depends on the type of ambulance carrying out the service. At the time of data collection, the mobile APH service in question was made up of nine ASBs, corresponding to the largest number of ambulances, whose team is made up only of the driver or firefighter and a nursing technician; five ASAs with a team made up of a doctor, nurse and firefighter or driver; and one rescue vehicle whose team is made up of a firefighter and a nursing technician. As you can see, the firefighter is the most representative, as he is present in all types of ambulance.

Of those interviewed, 46 (92%) said they had the full vaccination programme (3 doses) against the Hepatitis B virus, and four denied having the full vaccination programme. Of those not vaccinated (8.0%), two were firefighters, one a doctor and one a nurse. It's worth noting that of the unvaccinated professionals, three had been exposed to accidents with mbpc.

The HBV vaccine has a vaccine response of around 90 to 95 per cent in immunocompetent adults, and is widely recommended for all health professionals, in a series of three intramuscular doses; the second dose should be administered one month after the first and the third six months after the first dose (BRASIL, 2005).

Manetti et al. (2006) carried out a study of workers at a university hospital and found that 72.2 per cent were fully vaccinated against HBV; Balsamo and Felli (2006) carried out a similar study of hospital workers and found that 65 per cent were not fully vaccinated, citing a lack of time and opportunity as the reason for this situation.

Although the results of this study show a high rate of workers

It is estimated that around two million people in Brazil are infected with HBV, and around 700 million are developing liver cirrhosis or hepatocellular carcinoma" (GALIZZI FILHO, 2007, p. 35). The importance of vaccination against HBV can be seen in the data presented by the CDC (2003); the number of annual occupational notifications fell in the USA, surprisingly after the vaccine began to be used in 1982, from more than 10,000 cases in 1983 to less than 400 cases in 2001. With regard to hepatitis C, the number of infected healthcare workers is unknown; some studies estimate that 1% of these workers have evidence of hepatitis C virus infection (CDC, 2003). In view of this, there is a clear need for the correct and adequate use of PPE when carrying out procedures that could expose workers to the mbpc. To date, there is no specific vaccine or immunoglobulin available for hepatitis C prophylaxis.

Working in an emergency situation in a mobile APH has particular characteristics of the work environment itself. These particularities make workers more vulnerable to the risk of contamination by HBV and other microorganisms that cause serious or even fatal illnesses, through direct or indirect contact with blood, secretions, excretions and other body fluids.

Galizzi Filho (2007) warns that the environment, through its surfaces previously exposed to HBV-contaminated blood, is a source of contagion, since the virus can remain viable in these places for up to a week.

With regard to accidental exposure to mbpc, of the 50 interviewees in this study, 28 (56 per cent) reported having suffered some kind of accidental exposure.

Table 4 shows the distribution of the mobile APH team according to professional category and accidental exposure to mbpc.

Table 4 - Distribution of mobile prehospital care staff (n=50) according to professional category and accidental exposure to potentially contaminated biological material. Ribeirão Preto, 2007

Professional Category	Total	Accidental Exposure	
	n	*f*	%
Doctor	06	05	83,3
Nurse	08	06	75,0
Fireman	15	10	66,7
Nursing technician	12	05	41,7
Driver	09	02	22,2

It can be seen that among the professional categories with the highest proportion of accidents were doctors (83.3 per cent), followed by nurses (75 per cent), firefighters (66.7 per cent) and nursing technicians (41.6 per cent). The category that suffered the least accidental exposure to mbpc was ambulance drivers (22.2%).

Doctors, nurses, nursing technicians and firefighters are the professionals who have the most contact with patients, especially blood and other bodily fluids, in mobile APH. The driver, as well as driving the ambulance, most often assists the health team in removing the patient, but their contact time is shorter. It should not be forgotten that they also clean the vehicle, thus exposing themselves to biological risk.

Among the factors that interfere with the acquisition of occupational infection are the activities carried out by the professional, the sectors in which they work in the health service, the nature and frequency of exposure, the likelihood of exposure to biological agents, the worker's immunological response and the possibility of infection after certain exposure (GERBERDING, 1995).

Studies carried out on accidents involving sharps among healthcare professionals show that nursing staff are the ones who suffer the most accidents during their professional practice, with accidental exposure to sharps standing out (BASSO, 1999; BALSAMO; BARRIENTOS; ROSSI, 2000; BALSAMO, 2002; BREVIDELLI; CIANCIARULLO, 2002; SANTOS; ARAÚJO, 2003; RUIZ; BARBOSA; SOLER, 2004; MUROFUSE; MARZIALE; GEMELLI, 2005; BALSAMO; FELLI, 2006).

Takayanagui, Mendes and Dias (1993) refer to the nursing team as being the group most at risk of occupational exposure in the health area, due to the fact that their activities are predominantly manual, such as dressings, collecting materials for diagnostic tests, vaccinations, administering medicines, tracheal aspiration and body hygiene.

Bulhões (1998) highlights, among other reasons for the greater vulnerability of nursing staff to accidents, the fact that they carry out a greater volume of direct patient care with physical contact and perform a large number of invasive procedures.

As for the firefighters, 66.6 per cent of them were injured, a high rate given that they carry out very complex tasks in mobile APH. They are the ones who carry out the most effective extrication and extrication manoeuvres, among others, coming into direct contact with the victims, whose blood and other bodily fluids are abundant and in situations and locations that are often extremely difficult.

Table 5 shows the distribution of mbpc accidents according to the professional category of the mobile APH team and the type of accidental exposure.

Table 5 - Distribution of accidents (n=41) involving potentially contaminated biological material according to the professional category of the Mobile Pre-Hospital Care team and type of accidental exposure. Ribeirão Preto, 2007

Type of exhibition	Nursing Technician n = 12	Nurse n = 8	Doctor n = 6	Driver n = 9	Firefighter n = 15	TOTAL	
	f	*f*	*f*	*F*	*f*	*f*	%
Healthy skin	05	03	07	03	11	29	70,7
Percutaneous	02	02	00	00	03	07	17,1
Mucosa	01	01	00	00	01	03	7,3
Damaged skin	00	00	00	00	02	02	4,9
Total	08	06	07	03	17	41	100

Of the 50 workers interviewed, 28 reported accidental exposure to mbpc, totalling 41 accidents.

Of the total of 41 accidental exposures to mbpc, the majority (70.7 per cent) were to intact skin, followed by percutaneous accidents (17.1 per cent), exposure to mucous membranes (7.3 per cent) and, finally, exposure to damaged skin (4.9 per cent).

In the study carried out by Florêncio et al. (2003) on adherence to standard precautions, in which 44 professionals from the pre-hospital rescue team of the Goiás fire brigade took part, 12 of them had already had an accident at work with mbpc (27.3%); of those who had had an accident, five (41.7%) reported accidental exposure to blood or other body fluid on non-intact skin and four (33.3%)

on mucous membranes.

Another study on adherence to standard precautions by the mobile APH team in Belo Horizonte, Minas Gerais (LOPES et al. 2008), in which 238 professionals took part, found an incidence of (20.6%) accidents at work involving mbpc; of these, 49% were due to contact with bodily fluids on mucous membranes, (40.8%) due to handling sharp materials, and (10.2%) due to both.

Caixeta and Barbosa-Branco (2005) studied the occurrence of accidents at work involving biological material among health professionals, involving 570 subjects; those who reported the most accidents involving biological material were dental surgeons (64.3%), followed by doctors (47.8%) and nursing technicians (46%), while the lowest rate was for pharmacist-biochemists (17.6%); when considering all professionals, they observed that (86.5%) of all accidents involved percutaneous exposure, with the pharmacist-biochemist, nursing assistant, nursing assistant and dental surgeon categories standing out as those with the highest percentage of accidents; the categories with the highest percentage of accidental exposure through skin-mucous contact with potentially contaminated fluids were nurses (23.5%) and laboratory technicians (13.0%).

In recent years, various researchers (GIR; COSTA; SILVA, 1998; BRANDI; BENATTI; ALEXANDRE, 1998; ABREU; MAURO, 2000; BALSAMO; BARRIENTOS; ROSSI, 2000; SOUZA; VIANNA, 2000; BENATTI, 2001; TOMAZIN et al. 2001; CANINI et al., 2002; SARQUIS; FELLI, 2002; SÊCCO et al, 2003; NISHIDE; BENATTI, 2004; MARZIALE; NISHIMURA; FERREIRA, 2004; BARBOZA; SOLER; CIORLIA, 2004; RUIZ; BARBOSA; SOLER, 2004; MUROFUSE; MARZIALE; GEMELLI, 2005; BALSAMO; FELLI, 2006; MANETTI et al, 2006) have studied accidents involving mbpc in health institutions, especially hospitals and nursing teams, in recent years and have highlighted accidents involving sharps as the most common and, of course, the most worrying.

Exposure to biological risks can be increased in mobile APH due to the characteristics of the care provided, as stated by Mafra, et al. (2008), often in extremely complex situations, such as the accident scene, difficult-to-access locations, stress in the rapid handling of care and others.

In this study, when the subjects were asked during the interview if they had suffered any accidental exposure to mbpc, many answered in the negative. However, when asked if they had had any exposure to intact skin, a significant number said yes, but that they did not consider this type of exposure to be an accident.

Accidental exposure to intact skin generally refers to splashes and spillages of mbpc during procedures. Many professionals disregard this type of accident. The literature has not identified any reference to the transmission of disease due to accidents of this type, but it is worrying nonetheless. As Canalli (2008) points out, apparently intact skin can contain microlesions, often imperceptible, which can serve as a gateway to various types of infectious agents, including HIV, HVB and HVC.

It is believed that the high rate of accidental exposure to intact skin found in this study is mainly due to two situations. The first is the fact that the data was collected by interview, which enabled the researcher to confirm whether there had been any incidents of exposure to mbpc on intact skin, for those who did not mention this type of exposure. The second was due to the specific characteristics of the work of the mobile APH team, whose urgent/emergency care is most often carried out at the scene of the accident, with direct contact with the victim and the presence of blood and other body fluids; carrying out procedures in poorly lit places and in the moving ambulance, in limited space, among others.

Table 5 shows that doctors and drivers were only affected by accidental exposures to whole skin, while nursing technicians, nurses and firefighters were exposed to more than whole skin, such as percutaneous, damaged skin and mucous membranes.

Several studies involving health professionals show that nursing staff are the most frequently injured. Santos and Santos (2008) carried out a study of healthcare workers such as doctors, nurses, nursing technicians and assistants, cleaning service providers and students working in a University Hospital and found that the professional category most affected was the nursing assistant (81%), and that in (46.2%) of the accidents, the professionals did not use PPE or CPE - Collective Protection Equipment - when carrying out procedures. According to the CDC (2003), there were 57 confirmed cases in the United States of America of healthcare workers who seroconverted to HIV after accidental exposure at work, between 1985 and 2002. Of these, 26 developed AIDS; another 139 professionals reported HIV infection through alleged occupational exposure. Among the 57 workers infected with HIV, 24 were nurses and, among the suspected cases, 35 belonged to the same professional category. Two studies published in national journals on accidents with biological material obtained similar results: nursing staff were the most affected by accidents with biological material and punctures occurred in more than 80 per cent of these accidents (MUROFUSE et al., 2006).

On the other hand, in a study carried out by Machado (2006) at the occupational accidents clinic of the Hospital das Clínicas of the Ribeirão Preto Medical School, 602 accidents involving health professionals were reported between 2004 and 2005. In this study, the professional category most affected was nursing technicians, assistants and carers (31.2%), followed by doctors (23.4%), students (18.6%), nurses (8.5%), cleaning and laundry service assistants and servants (6.8%), dentists (3.3%), laboratory technicians and assistants (1.8%), biologists and biomedical professionals (1%), pharmacists (0.3%), and others (2.8%). Among the source patients (2.3%) were seropositive for HBV (HBsAg), (6.5%) for HCV and (8%) for HIV. There was no seroconversion to HBV, HCV or HIV. Table 6 shows the distribution of exposure to mbpc in the mobile APH team according to the type of care provided.

Table 6 - Distribution of accidental exposures to potentially contaminated biological material (n=41) in the mobile Pre-Hospital Care team according to type of care. Ribeirão Preto, 2007

Type of Service	Grand total		Exposure to mbpc	
	f	%	*f*	%
Mobile APH on motorways	40	80	37	90,2
Mobile APH in Urban Areas	10	20	04	9,8
Grand total	50	100	41	100

The majority of accidental exposures occurred during roadside assistance.

The justification for these figures can possibly be attributed to the difference in the types of service, the one that serves the urban area and the one that operates on the motorways.

The mobile APH that operates on the motorways provides care almost exclusively for traumas resulting from traffic accidents along the road network, which generally cause serious victims.

The type of ambulance used for mobile APH on motorways has a number of characteristics

These include: the presence of extrication devices; fire extinguishers; PPE for firefighting and for accidents involving dangerous products; tarpaulins for the care of multiple victims; ropes; chairs; carabiners, among others, for rescue at height. This structure is designed to cater for different situations, such as the handling and treatment of multiple victims, hostile situations such as victims trapped in ironwork or thrown over cliffs, among others, and who consequently have injuries with a large volume of blood, other bodily fluids and dirt.

All these dynamics demand a great deal of technical-scientific skill, agility, self-control and confidence on the part of the mobile APH professional working on motorways to deal with emergency situations and physical and emotional stress. The word agility is commonly used in urgent and emergency services, but this dynamic must not negatively interfere with the quality of the service provided and the use of PPE; even with all the stress of the situation, care protocols and biosafety standards must be followed correctly.

Stress imbued with the need to act quickly inhibits the ability to reflect and consequently to assess potential risks. Exaggerated self-confidence can also be an aggravating factor and become an element of occupational risk, especially among more experienced professionals in the field, who often believe that biosecurity measures are unnecessary (BIOSECURITY... 2007).

Table 7 shows the distribution of the types of accidents among the mobile APH team according to the variables: place affected, activity performed and time of accident. Table 7 - Distribution of the types of accidents among the Mobile Pre-Hospital Care team according to the variables: place affected, activity performed and time of care. Ribeirão Preto, 2008

Variables	Percutaneous accident *f*	Full skin contact *f*	Contact with damaged skin *f*	Mucosal contact *f*	Total *f*	Total %
Site affected						
Forearm	01	16	0	0	17	41,5
Hand	01	7	01	0	09	21,9
Arm	02	06	01	0	09	21,9
Face	0	05	0	0	05	12,2
Thigh	01	03	0	0	04	9,8
Finger	02	0	0	0	02	4,9
Eyes	0	0	0	02	02	4,9
Mouth	0	0	0	02	02	4,9
Neck	0	02	0	0	02	4,9
Abdomen	0	01	0	0	01	2,4
Activity carried out						
Immobilisation procedure	0	16	0	0	16	39,0
Extraction procedure	03	04	01	01	09	21,9
Physical examination	0	06	0	0	06	14,6
Tracheal intubation procedure	0	02	0	01	03	7,3
After inserting the needle into the patient	03	0	0	0	03	7,3
Cleaning mbpc	0	01	0	01	02	4,9
Ambulance check	01	0	0	0	01	2,4
Resuscitation						
Basic cardiopulmonary	0	0	01	0	01	2,4
Time of service						
With a patient in the ambulance	04	14	01	02	21	51,2
With a patient at the scene of the accident	02	15	01	01	19	46,3
With a patient in hospital	01	0	0	0	01	2,4

The most affected sites in the percutaneous accident were: forearm (17), arm (9) and hand (9).

Machado et al. (1992); Tomazin et al. (2001); Sêcco et al. (2003); Morufuse; Marziale;

Gemelli (2005), in studies on accidental exposures in nursing staff with mbpc, point to the fingers and hands as being the most affected topographies, with rates ranging from (74%) to (86.4%).

Studies carried out with undergraduate nursing, medical and dental students also confirm that the fingers and hands are the most affected regions, with rates ranging from 72.7 per cent to 93.2 per cent (KITAYAMA; MARINGOLO, 2000; SCOTTI, AGUILERA; SILVA, 2002; REIS; GIR; CANINI, 2004; CANALLI, 2008).

In the studies carried out on nursing staff and undergraduate students, there was no mention of the forearm as a site of accidental exposure to mbpc. It is understandable that the forearm is the most frequently exposed area for mobile APH workers, followed by the hand and arm, as initial care is predominantly manual; involves analysing the condition(s) of the patient(s) at the scene, transporting the patient from the scene to the ambulance, support procedures/maintaining the patient's life, not to mention the situations of extricating the victim(s) from hardware, transporting the victim(s) in places that are difficult to access, which expose them to contact with mbpc.

This situation can be better understood by looking at the activity that was being carried out when the accidental exposures occurred and the time of care. In terms of activities, accidental exposures occurred when the following procedures were carried out: immobilisation (16); extrication (9); physical examination (06) and post-insertion of a needle into the patient (3). Accidental exposure occurred when the patient was being cared for in the ambulance (21) at the scene of the accident (19) and in hospital (01).

Blood was considered the most frequent biological material with 33 exposures (85.0%) among the total number of accidents reported by the mobile APH team, followed by vomit with seven (17.1%). It should be noted that blood is the biological material most at risk of transmitting HIV, HBV and HCV (BRASIL, 2005).

Balsamo and Felli (2006) and Manetti et al. (2006) estimated the involvement of blood in (44.85%) and (73%), respectively, of exposures to cGMP suffered by hospital workers.

In studies carried out with nurses, Nhamba (2004) points to blood and blood derivatives as the main cause of mbpc accidents.

Table 8 shows the distribution of situations favouring accidental exposure (n=41) according to mobile APH team professionals.

Table 8 - Distribution of situations favouring accidental exposure according to mobile prehospital care team professionals (n=28). Ribeirão Preto, 2007

Favourable situations	*f*	%
Emergency	13	46,4
Patient agitation	08	28,6
Rescue operations	07	25,0
Distraction	06	21,4
Stress	05	17,9
Large volumes of biological material	04	14,3
Multiple victims	03	10,7
Hurry	02	7,1
Unsuitable materials	02	7,1
Lighting	01	3,6
Little experience	01	3,6
Restricted space	01	3,6
Technical difficulty	01	3,6

According to the professionals from the mobile APH team who suffered accidents, the situations that most favoured accidental exposure to mbpc were: emergency (13), followed by agitation (8), rescue operations (7), distraction (6), large volume of mbpc (4) and stress (5).

When analysing other studies carried out on nursing workers, it can be seen that similar situations contributed to the occurrence of accidents. In the study by Tomazin et al. (2001), the injured nursing staff mentioned rushing (18.5 per cent) and carelessness (14.8 per cent) as factors related to accidents, but also (14.8 per cent) stated that there were no factors. Nhamba (2004) in a study carried out with nursing staff in Angola - Africa found that (37.7%) of the research subjects did not mention any cause, (26%) cited the emergency and (24.3%) distraction, among the causes that favoured the accident. Nishide, Benatti and Alexandre (2004), in a study of accidents that occurred among intensive care unit nursing staff, found inattention (17%), not wearing PPE (13%) and haste (13%) as possible causes.

Among healthcare workers in a hospital, Balsamo and Felli (2006) found the most frequent causes to be: inappropriate use of the technique (25 per cent), chance (19.64 per cent), inattention (16.7 per cent) and haste (12.5 per cent).

Among undergraduate nursing, medical and dental students, the situations favouring accidental exposure to mbpc were diverse. In the study by Canalli (2008), the situations mentioned by nursing students were: not using PPE (49.1%), inattention (45%), stress (25.4%), haste (25.4), nervousness (21.9%), pressure from the teacher (20%) and inexperience (20%). Ribeiro (2005) listed the following causes of accidents among dental students: distraction, haste, stress, tiredness and inexperience. In the study by Scotti, Aguilera and Silva (2002), most of the nursing students mentioned fear or pressure from the supervising teacher when carrying out activities as factors that can contribute to accidents; this fact favoured some students not reporting accidents. According to the study by Reis et al. (2004), medical students reported a lack of care (45.3%) and inexperience (30.9%) as situations that favoured accidents. Ribeiro (2005), when carrying out a study with dental students, found that distraction, haste, stress, tiredness and inexperience favoured accidental exposure to mbpc.

When analysing the situations favouring accidental exposure to mbpc mentioned by undergraduate nursing, medicine and dentistry students, and the situations mentioned by health professionals in general and nursing professionals in hospital institutions and also in mobile APH, many points in common can be seen: stress/nervousness/fear; distraction/inattention/carelessness/lack of care; inexperience/inadequate act when carrying out the technique; not using PPE; haste/agitation/rush/emergency/pressure.

In addition to all these factors common to healthcare professionals, mobile APH workers face other favourable situations: rescue operations and the large volume of mbpc, which can make them more vulnerable to accidental exposure to mbpc than other healthcare professionals.

In the context of the work of the mobile APH team, an important point to highlight is the stress factor in their daily work.

Occupational stressors vary according to the activities and can be physical, chemical, biological and social in nature, resulting from intrinsic or extrinsic factors in the individual (BACHION et al., 1998). In a study on stress in a military pre-hospital rescue team, Aguiar et al. (2000) found that rescuers suggest a simplistic view of what stress is, explaining the phenomenon as physical and mental tiredness and nervousness. They pointed out that it is difficult for them to define stress, but that they recognise stress when they feel it. The authors identified the fear of the unknown, the violence of the scenes, and organisational and personal demands as sources of tension and anxiety. With regard to fear of the unknown, the sources listed by the first responders were the sounding of the siren, travelling to the scene and always being on the alert; with regard to the violence of the scenes, they were the involvement of children, the elderly and family members, and the accident scene itself; and with regard to institutional and personal demands, they described the large number of incidents, the extensive workload, obligations to be skilful and quick, job dissatisfaction and the search for perfectionism.

According to Bachion (1998), the alarm reaction is the first stage of the stress reaction, which mobilises organic defence forces, involving signs of tachycardia, sweating, irritability and fatigue; by repeatedly entering this phase of stress, over time the person can enter the other phase of stress, i.e. resistance and exhaustion, leading to health problems.

For Yanes et al (1993), among the various situations that can cause stress in human beings, one of the most important is stress at work, given that the way they live and work determines how they fall ill. Various diseases such as hypertension, peptic ulcers, acute myocardial infarction, alcoholism, among others, are attributed to stress (BACHION, 1998).

Given the above, it can certainly be inferred that stress is an extremely important factor that favours accidental exposure not only to biological risk, but to all other occupational risks.

An important piece of data that deserves to be evaluated is that of those who do not mentioned no cause as favourable (8%) for accidental exposure to mbpc. This behaviour can be interpreted as: these professionals trivialising accidental exposure to mbpc; believing it to be inherent to the work process they perform and therefore not perceiving any predisposing cause; or lack of knowledge/lack of preparation on the part of the professionals.

Table 9 shows the distribution of the research subjects according to the following variables: use of PPE, behaviour in the affected area, post-exposure behaviour and opening of a CAT.

Table 9 - Distribution of accidents with potentially contaminated material (n=41) among workers on the mobile Pre-Hospital Care team according to the variables: use of Personal Protective Equipment, behaviour in the affected area, behaviour after exposure, and opening of a Work Accident Report. Ribeirão Preto, 2007

Variables	Percutaneous accident	Full skin contact	Contact with damaged skin	Mucosal contact	Total	
	f	*f*	*f*	*f*	*f*	%
Use of PPE						
Latex gloves (procedures)	02	23	01	0	26	63,4
Rubber glove	0	02	0	0	02	4,9
Leather / vaqueta glove	0	03	0	0	03	7,3
Goggles	0	10	0	0	10	24,4
Face mask	0	06	0	0	06	14,6
Denim overalls	06	29	01	03	39	95,1
Fire approach clothing and helmet	01	0	01	0	02	4,9
Long boots	05	27	02	03	37	90,2
Conduct in the affected area						
Washed with soap and water	04	12	01	01	18	43,9
Used antiseptic	02	15	0	0	17	41,5
Used only water	01	0	01	01	03	7,3
No behaviour	0	02	0	01	03	7,3
Post-exposure behaviour						
Had a medical consultation	04	03	02	03	12	29,3
Serological tests (HIV, HBV, HCV) carried out	04	0	01	02	07	25,0

Needed Prophylaxis - HIV	01	0	0	0	01	2,4
Needed Prophylaxis - HBV	0	0	0	01	01	2,4
He judged it unnecessary	03	26	0	0	29	70,7
Opening a CAT						
Yes	04	02	01	02	09	21,9
No	03	27	01	01	32	78,1

As for the use of PPE, all of them reported wearing suitable clothing for the job, i.e. denim overalls (95.1%) or specific fire approach clothing and a helmet (4.1%); 90.2% reported wearing high-top boots (their own purchase). Latex/procedure gloves were used by the majority (63.4%). The other most commonly used PPE was goggles (24.4%) and a face mask (14.6). Leather gloves (7.3%) and rubber gloves (4.9%) were also used.

Denim overalls are compulsory in the mobile APH service; there is no possibility of not wearing them, their use goes beyond protection and also serves to identify the professional to the company and the public. Denim overalls are only dispensed with when there is a need for special protection with other types of clothing, such as in the event of a fire, for example. Although long boots are considered PPE and their use is recommended by the company, they were not supplied by the company at the time of data collection. A few professionals from the mobile APH team mentioned during the interview that they didn't wear high-top boots because they were uncomfortable, opting instead for trainers/shoes.

Procedural gloves should be worn whenever there is direct contact with the patient; the use of a face mask and goggles is recommended to protect the mucous membranes of the eyes, nose and mouth when carrying out procedures and activities that could generate splashes and/or sprays of blood and other body fluids, secretions and excretions (SEIDEL et al., 2007).

The long sleeves serve as a protective barrier against biological fluids, mechanical or physical-chemical agents. During the interviews, it was observed that the majority of professionals were not wearing the sleeves of their overalls and some of them verbalised that they didn't use them during victim care, justifying the fact that they were uncomfortable and hot. It is worth remembering that among the body regions, the forearm was the one most exposed to mbpc, which demonstrates the importance of uniform sleeves in protecting not only against biological risks, but also against other occupational risks.

In the study by Florêncio et al. (2003), it was found that although the respondents used procedure gloves, masks and goggles during risk situations, observation revealed that procedure gloves were the only measure used.

In a study on adherence to SP by the mobile APH team in Belo Horizonte - MG, Lopes et al. (2008) found that the greater the knowledge, the more positive the attitudes; doctors and nurses showed greater knowledge and were better able to adopt standard precautions than drivers and nursing assistants/technicians.

Mafra et al. (2008), when studying nurses' perceptions of the importance of using PPE for biological risks in a mobile APH service, concluded that they realise its importance and are aware of the risks to which they are exposed; however, this perception is not enough to use it in everyday practice.

PPE is essential to promote safety at work, but studies involving healthcare workers in general, nurses, firefighters and mobile APH teams (BRIVIDELLI; CINCIARULLO, 2002; FLORÊNCIO et al., 2003; NICHIATA et al., 2005; LOPES et al., 2008; MAFRA et al., 2008) indicate that many professionals are resistant to using it.

In fact, the statement made by the various authors cited above can be confirmed in the words of one of the interviewees in this study, who did not wear protective glasses, believing that the corrective lenses used would have the same effect, despite seeing blood splatter on his lenses after seeing patients.

According to Mafra et al. (2008), adopting safe practices to prevent accidents involves factors intrinsic to the subject, addictions, the will of those involved and their knowledge.

You can also add the involvement of extrinsic factors at the institution/company, such as the availability of quality PPE and CPE in sufficient quantity, proper waste management involving mbpc, among others.

As for the immediate action taken at the site exposed to the mbpc, the majority (43.9%) washed with soap and water, which is recommended by the CDC (2003); (41.5%) used antiseptics, which is not ruled out, as the literature review did not find any studies on its benefits. It is worth noting that there were situations in which only water was used for cleaning (7.3%) and also those exposed to mbpc who did not take any action (7.3%). Proper and immediate cleaning of the area with soap and water is essential for removing the infecting agent.

The most frequent course of action after accidental exposure was to seek medical advice (29.3%) followed by HBV, HCV and HIV serological tests (25%); the majority (70.7%) did not open a CAT.

When comparing tables 5 and 8, it is clear that in three percutaneous accidents no medical consultations were carried out, nor were serologies for HBV, HCV and HIV, as there were a total of seven percutaneous accidents and only in four were medical consultations and serologies carried out. In the case of accidental exposures to mucous membranes (3) and damaged skin (2), it is clear that medical consultations and serological tests were carried out in both cases, as the numbers in both tables coincide.

CATs were opened for nine (21.9%) accidental exposures. Considering that there were a total of 12 accidents with a potential risk of contamination, three accidents were not reported.

In the event of accidental exposure to mbpc, it is essential to immediately go to a health centre that is available 24 hours a day, designated for comprehensive care in this situation. If possible, take the source patient or their blood with you for serological tests, with the consent of the patient or their guardian, in writing and with two witnesses, as part of the mbpc accident protocol. Each service must present a contingency plan and train its professionals to provide emergency care in the event of accidents involving mbpc. The severity of the exposure should be analysed and appropriate follow-up given, if possible within the first two hours of exposure, especially HIV prophylaxis through antiretroviral drugs (BRASIL, 2005a). In this case, it is the injured person who is facing an emergency and should be immediately referred for the necessary care.

During the interview, all the professionals from the mobile APH team taking part in the research (n=50) were asked about the existence of rules for the prevention and control of accidents with biological material and the protocol for behaviour after accidental exposure to mbpc in the service. They were also asked about training in occupational risks in mobile APH and PPE during their induction period at the company.

It was found that 94 per cent of professionals were aware of the rules for preventing accidents with mbpc and (96 per cent) of the protocol for post-exposure conduct to mbpc; (96 per cent) reported having received training on occupational risks in mobile APH, and 96 per cent on PPE.

Although the majority of the workers in the mobile APH team said they were aware of the rules for preventing accidents involving mbpc, the protocol for post-exposure behaviour towards mbpc, and that they had received training on occupational risks in mobile APH and on PPE, some stopped using it, as can be seen in Table 9, page 101, when they didn't open a CAT in the event of an accident involving mbpc.

PPE is essential to ensure minimum safety standards for workers at work, but many still trivialise the conduct recommended for accident prevention, in this particular case for the mbpc, believing in their possible invulnerability to accidents and contamination by biological agents.

Adopting the practice of using PPE and preventive measures against biological risks will only be successful when each professional is made aware of its importance and recognises it as an act of individual and collective responsibility.

According to Costa (2003), biosafety must be understood not only as a process of acquiring skills or concepts, but must be transmitted through an educational process that transcends training. Education implies sharing actions and conceiving agents as subjects of learning, involving individuals as a whole, considering their differences and singularities (MOREIRA, 2002).

Table 10 shows the distribution of responses from the professionals in the mobile APH team, according to the variables cleaning of the ambulance, disinfection of materials, packaging and disposal of biological waste.

With regard to cleaning ambulances, all (100 per cent) of the professionals said that they were cleaned with soap and water; (98 per cent) said that they used sodium hypochlorite; and 28 per cent said that they used other types of solutions, such as 70 per cent alcohol and other general household cleaning solutions.

As for cleaning/disinfecting material, (96%) reported using soap and water, (96%) sodium hypochlorite and (4%) glutaraldehyde. The study in question did not ask about the concentration used of these solutions, but it is worth noting that the product should be used correctly, according to the supplier's instructions.

Cleaning, i.e. the removal of dirt in order to maintain the hygiene of the ambulance, should follow the same procedure adopted in health institutions, and the use of soap and water is recommended. All materials, stretchers and other items should be removed from the ambulance and cleaned as often as possible. This routine should last approximately two hours (SKOVGAARD, 1989).

The professionals involved in this process must wear PPE (gloves, waterproof apron and goggles) to clean the vehicle (HOEFEL, n.d.).

Table 10 - Distribution of responses from mobile Pre-Hospital Care team professionals (n=50) according to the variables cleaning of the ambulance, disinfection of materials, packaging and disposal of biological waste. Ribeirão Preto, 2007

Variables	**Yes**		**No**		**Don't know**	
	f	%	*f*	%	*f*	%

How to clean an ambulance						
Use of soap and water	50	100	0	0	0	0
Use of sodium hypochlorite	49	98,0	01	2,0	0	0
Use of other substances	14	26,0	0	0	0	0
How to clean/disinfect materials						
Use of soap and water	48	96,0	01	2,0	01	2,0
Use of sodium hypochlorite	48	96,0	01	2,0	01	2,0
Use of glutaraldehyde	02	4,0	47	94,0	01	2,0
Form of packaging						
Sharps in ordinary rubbish	0	0	50	100	0	0
Sharps in rigid-walled rubbish bins	44	88,0	06	12,0	0	0
Other biological materials in ordinary rubbish bins	05	10,0	45	90,0	0	0
Sharps in plastic containers	43	86,0	07	14,0	0	0
Final disposal of solid waste						
In the rubbish bin	0	0	49	98,0	01	2,0
In hospital waste	49	98,0	0	0	01	2,0
Final disposal of liquid waste						
Rainwater	08	16,0	30	60,0	12	24,0
Trench	*27*	54,0	0	0	*23*	46,0

After cleaning/disinfecting the vehicle, the mattress and plastic-lined pillows should be sanitised with soap and water to help remove adhered dirt (SKOVGAARD, 1989).

Regarding the use of other substances to clean ambulances and materials (26 per cent), they mentioned 70 per cent alcohol and a general-purpose cleaning solution for the home (composition: sodium aquyl benzene sulphanate, ethoxylated alcohol, sequestering aids, fragrance and water).

All semi-critical or non-critical equipment or articles that come into contact with healthy skin and/or healthy mucous membranes that are not contaminated with blood, fluids or biological liquids require low or medium-level cleaning or disinfection to guarantee their quality for multiple use, or to be carefully disposed of as hospital waste. Critical articles, materials that cross the skin and/or mucous membrane barrier, require sterilisation (BRASIL, 1994b).

Of those interviewed, 56 per cent reported not having a purge in their service, but a tank for cleaning materials. During the interview, it was mentioned that the same tank was used for a variety of purposes, such as sanitising kitchen utensils and personal hygiene.

With regard to the form of packaging used for sharps, all (100%) of the professionals said they didn't dispose of it in ordinary rubbish, while 88% said they disposed of it in appropriate rigid-walled cardboard rubbish. With regard to other waste contaminated by biological materials, such as gauze, cotton wool, among others, 90% said they did not use ordinary rubbish. An interesting fact is that 86% reported disposing of sharps in improvised plastic containers with lids, which is not recommended.

Mobile APH team workers reported having difficulty disposing of sharps when invasive procedures are carried out at the scene of an accident; they are taken manually to the appropriate box fixed to the vehicle for disposal.

Sharps should be disposed of in appropriate bins immediately after use to avoid accidental exposure (GARNER, 1996).

As can be seen in Table 7, page 107, among the moments when accidental exposure with mbpc occurred among professionals in the mobile APH team, (7.3%) reported "after insertion of needle in patient". According to Souza (2001) the handling of sharps after use has been responsible for a large proportion of percutaneous accidents.

With regard to solid waste, (98%) of the professionals reported disposing of it in hospital waste, of these (8%) reported handing it over to another ambulance and then disposing of it in the hospital and (2%) didn't know.

Infectious waste can pose a potential risk to public health and the environment. Therefore, it must be packaged in a white plastic bag with specifications in accordance with NBR 7500/94, labelled with the infectious substance symbol, placed in a bin with a lid that closes it hermetically; its volume must not exceed 2/3 of the bin's capacity (RIBEIRO FILHO, 2000).

As for the disposal of liquid waste, 54 per cent said it went down the drain and the rest (46 per cent) couldn't say where it went. According to (8 per cent) of the professionals, the water used to wash the ambulances flows into the rainwater. These procedures should be reviewed, as they can cause serious damage to the health of the population and the environment.

When asked about the factors that favour accidental exposure to biological risks in mobile APH, 92% of the professionals presented one or more risk factors. The answers were categorised according to their similarities (Chart 1).

Categories	Risk factors
Accident site	- Scene of the accident - Victim trapped in hardware - Decarceration - Curious onlookers - Flow of vehicles
User service	- Agitated victim - Emergency/urgent situation - Large volume of blood/body fluids
Physical space	- Reduced space to carry out actions - Ambulance not sanitised -Lack of space and organisation inside the ambulance
Environmental factors	- Rain - Wind/storm - Extreme temperatures (heat/cold) - Places that are difficult to access (slopes, rough terrain, etc.) - Poor lighting (night service)
Experience in the field	-Lack of practical skills/lack of experience -Lack of training in mobile APH -Non-use/incorrect use of PPE
Biopsycho-emotional factor	- Stress - Nervousness - Emotional instability in the face of the situation - Fear of doing the wrong thing - Lack of team integration - Lack of self-confidence - Lack of physical preparation/conditioning - Lack of concentration - Involvement of children and the elderly in the scene - Tiredness - Sleep

Chart 1 - Factors that favoured accidental exposure to biological risks in mobile prehospital care, according to professionals from the mobile prehospital care team.

Chart 1 shows that some of the risk factors mentioned by the Mobile APH Team professionals are no different from those mentioned by other healthcare workers, such as: not using/using PPE incorrectly; stress; nervousness; tiredness; sleep. The vast majority of risk factors mentioned by mobile APH team professionals are specific, inherent to mobile APH work.

This finding leads us to recognise that preventing biological risks in mobile APH requires general measures applicable to other healthcare sectors, and specific prevention measures for the risk factors inherent in mobile APH.

As measures to prevent mbpc accidents, the professionals from the mobile APH team made several suggestions, which were grouped together taking into account their similarities:

- Use PPE correctly;
- Increase the number of specific trainings in mobile APH;
- Uniform with waterproof fabric and no detachable sleeves;
- Suitable gloves, longer and more resistant;
- Implement the use of long-sleeved plastic aprons;
- Greater awareness among professionals of biological risks;
- Company demand for the use of masks and goggles;
- Improve the quality of training;
- Encourage attendance at training sessions;
- Build drainage at the base of motorways;
- Emotional support for the company's mobile APH team professionals;
- Implement the use of specific materials for invasive procedures with safety devices;
- Have a portable container for storing waste while still at the scene;
- Creation of CIPA.

At the end of each interview, the interviewee (E) was given the opportunity to make any comments if they wished; of the total of 50 participants, 12 (24 per cent) made the following comments:

- "Improve the flow of information regarding the post-exposure care protocol." (E1)

- "It's important for colleagues to attend training sessions on PPE and risks in mobile APH, which should be repeated every six (6) months. A protocol (steps) should be created to record the presence of mbpc accidents. The use of an N95 mask should be implemented in the PPE routine". (E2)

- "Convincing professionals of the occupational risks they are exposed to when they don't wear gloves or goggles." (E3)

- "I would like to have lectures/training on the risks of accidents with biological material." (E4)

- "Having a temporary place at the operational bases to store infected materials with biological material until they are delivered to the hospital, so as not to leave them in the ambulance for too long." (E5)

- "Improving the internal layout of the ambulance (physical space), facilitating the flow of traffic and reducing the risk of accidents involving mbpc." (E6)

- "Tell colleagues to be more careful when handling sharps after use. The team usually puts the needle in the mattress, because access to the proper container is difficult, I prefer to put it on the floor and step on it." (E7)

- "Everyone should ask if the victim has any health problems. There should be more training on infectious diseases such as tuberculosis, ways of transmission and aseptic care." (E8)

- "The PPE offered by the company is suitable for the work he does." (E9)

- "There are situations in which the PPE doesn't help, it's not enough, for example: heavy-duty gloves.

procedure does not adequately protect the professional in the presence of sharps infected with biological materials". (E10)

- "My life depends on PPE". (Eli)

- "With regard to the tank for cleaning the bases on the motorways, it should be in a more appropriate place and not used for various purposes." (E12)

5.1 Suggested strategies for preventing and controlling accidents involving mbpc in mobile APH

The proposals for strategies to prevent and control accidents involving mbpc in mobile APH were based on the results of this study, suggestions from the professionals on the mobile APH team who took part in the study, a literature review, the author's experience of mobile APH and the supervisor's experience of occupational accidents involving mbpc.

The suggested proposals were categorised into specific and general measures. The specific ones refer to measures for mobile APH and the general measures are those applied to all health professionals, regardless of their area of expertise.

5.1.2 Specific measures for mobile APH

Choosing a mobile APH vehicle that is suitable in terms of internal space and stability is fundamental for the safety and comfort of the team and the patient. Vehicles for emergency medical care and rescue must comply with NBR 14561/2000 (ABNT, 2008), which sets out the minimum conditions required for the design, construction and performance of vehicles for emergency medical care and rescue.

It is important to note the existence of materials for the structural reinforcement of the ambulance in order to protect the team and the client in the event of a collision/rollover, as well as reinforcement to receive cabinets and equipment.

The vehicle intended for mobile APH on motorways must take into account certain particularities, such as: transporting more than one victim at the same time; the presence of equipment such as de-escalators; fire extinguishers; PPE for firefighting, de-escalation and acting in the presence of dangerous products; tarpaulins for assisting multiple victims; ropes; chairs; carabiners, among others, for rescue at height. This requires a detailed study of how to accommodate all the items so as not to overload the ambulance in terms of both weight and space.

Vehicles must receive routine preventive maintenance, which is essential to ensure the safety of users and the mobile APH team, as well as good performance.

The interior of the ambulance must be lined with waterproof, washable material, with rounded corners to ensure safety and ease of cleaning and disinfection. It should be completely sealed so that water and waste (blood, vomit, etc.) do not penetrate through the gaps and settle below the panelling. It is recommended that the ambulance floor be covered in a non-slip material that seamlessly covers the entire floor and the skirting board by 10 centimetres or more. The holes in the floor for fixing the seats and stretchers must also be sealed to prevent liquids from passing under the covering. Seams and finishes must be glued with a dense, paste-like polyurethane adhesive with good adhesion to different types of materials to prevent vibrations and temperature variations.

It is common to use naval plywood to level the original floor of the ambulance, but water and debris can seep through, damaging the wood and the original floor of the vehicle. It is suggested that a rubberised material be used to cover the floor, as it is non-slip and outperforms the others in terms of durability, impermeability, ease of cleaning and replacement.

Wall and ceiling coverings can be made of fibreglass, injected material or formicated marine plywood, the latter being the most suitable because it is more resistant. Places susceptible to collisions with stretchers or other heavy materials should be protected with stainless steel plates, as they are more resistant and easier to clean.

For the safety of the team members, the vehicle must have three-point seat belts to ensure their immobilisation in impact situations/car crashes.

Gas cylinders and fire extinguishers must be restrained with belts and suitable structures so that they do not move on impact.

Due to the limited space inside the ambulance, the internal walls must be free so that the team's professionals can move around easily during assistance and do not collide with objects installed in this space.

The mobile APH service must provide a suitable place for the exclusive cleaning and decontamination of used and/or soiled materials. Water derived from the process of cleaning contaminated materials should be subjected to a specific decontamination treatment process before being disposed of in the common sewer, in order to minimise environmental contamination (SILVA, 2004).

There also needs to be a dedicated area for preparing and storing clean and/or sterile material. If the service cannot accommodate this type of structure, another strategy must be devised to control the situation, such as hiring an outsourced service to carry out the work or using predominantly disposable materials.

For cleaning dirt to maintain the hygiene of ambulances, we recommend using soap and water or a neutral detergent.

Surfaces with blood, body fluids, secretions, excretions and/or other mbpc materials should be cleaned and disinfected using a 1:10 solution of sodium hypochlorite-bleach solution, which has great microbial action and rapid effect. On the other hand, it has corrosive properties, is inactivated by organic material and is unstable, so its use is limited to rubberised materials that are subject to corrosion and in the presence of organic material.

After cleaning the vehicle, a cloth soaked in 70% alcohol should be used to help remove grease, eliminate pathogenic microorganisms and aid quick drying, except on acrylics.

Mattresses and pillows lined with plastic should also be sanitised with 70% alcohol to help remove adhered dirt when soap and water cannot be used.

Sheets and pillowcases should be changed for each patient and sent for hospital reprocessing.

Professionals involved in the cleaning/disinfection process must wear gloves, an impermeable apron and goggles.

Ambulances must be cleaned on washable surfaces with drains. The water from washing the ambulances must be disposed of down the drain.

Waste collection should be selective, as it not only promotes worker safety but also reduces costs. The rigid-walled, waterproof container for the disposal of infectious materials should be located in a strategic, well-fixed place to facilitate the disposal of sharps and mbpc. If invasive procedures take place at the scene of the accident, a smaller, rigid-walled, impermeable container should be available for the disposal of sharps and MBPC, to avoid accidental exposure, either at this location or on the route between the scene of the accident and the ambulance, where there is a specific rubbish bin for the disposal of these materials.

When hiring professionals for the mobile APH team, the guidelines set out in CFM RESOLUTION No. 1,596/2000 should be followed, which indicates the necessary profile of the mobile APH team (BRASIL, 2000).

Training for professionals working in mobile APH should be based on Ordinance 2048/2002 (BRASIL, 2002), which sets out the content and minimum workload required for each professional category.

Training must be given before the worker takes up the job and then on an ongoing basis, according to NR 32 (BRASIL, 2005b).

It is proposed that mobile APH services have technical support from the SEESMT in order to control and record accidents at work. Risk mapping is also important.

Specific personal protective equipment (PPE) must be used according to the needs of the service.

We suggest evaluating the cost-benefit of more resistant, longer gloves with a better anatomical shape, which adapt better to the hands and forearm, providing greater dexterity and safety for mobile APH professionals.

It is important that after using the protective gloves, they are discarded immediately so as not to contaminate utensils such as clipboards, cupboards, doors, etc.

Hand hygiene should always be carried out before and after any procedure, including sequential procedures on the same patient, involving direct contact with the patient or indirect contact with potentially contaminated materials. In mobile APH, this care often becomes unfeasible when there are no resources available for this procedure, such as at the scene of the accident. When it is not possible to sanitise hands with soap and water, use 70% alcohol gel. Alcohol solutions do not rule out the need to sanitise hands with soap and water, when possible. It is recommended that mobile APH team members always wash their hands with soap and water when they return to their service and/or hospital institutions.

In view of the high level of exposure to noise generated by horns and sirens, professionals in the mobile APH team should undergo annual preventive audiometry tests. The use of hearing protection is important and should be part of the PPE, along with long-sleeved overalls, long boots, an N95 mask, goggles and gloves, which should be provided in quantity and quality by the company/institution.

Keep the necessary forms and materials for reporting occupational accidents inside the mobile APH vehicle, as a facilitator for aggregating data and taking blood if necessary (with the informed consent of the patient or guardian).

Have antiretroviral drugs (two reverse transcriptase inhibitors) available in the ambulance for emergency use in the event of an indication for HIV prophylaxis. This initial prophylaxis does not rule out the need to continue it in order to complete the programme, if necessary, and for this the injured person should go to the designated place to complete the treatment.

An extremely important aspect is not to keep any flammable product inside the ambulance (e.g. ether, benzine) to avoid explosions when using medical gauze, especially.

5.1.3 General measures

a) Individual

Every health professional needs to be effectively integrated into their company's/institution's occupational accident prevention programme, taking part in training, evaluating and making suggestions for improvement.

Carrying out the full vaccination programme against HBV and other indicated vaccines is the responsibility of each professional. You should not wait for the company/institution to charge you.

When necessary, post-exposure prophylaxis should be started as soon as possible, within the first two hours after the accident. The maximum time limit for starting post-exposure prophylaxis with antiretrovirals is up to 72 hours after the accident (BRASIL, 2006).

Adoption of simple measures that minimise accidental exposure, such as:

- adherence to Standard Precautions;
- proper use of Personal Protective Equipment (PPE);
- Contaminated needles and other sharps must not be bent or recapped;
- mbpc should be disposed of immediately in rigid-walled, impermeable containers and replaced when they reach two thirds of their capacity;
- report the accident as soon as possible to the company/institution where you work and seek specific assistance to prevent possible damage to your health; if there is no assistance on site, seek assistance at the nearest place of reference, in order to guarantee adequate follow-up;
- avoid unnecessary handling of sharps and mbpc;

b) Institutional (employers)

- Adopt a structured biosafety programme and implement appropriate strategies to prevent accidents and minimise occupational risks in the event of accidental exposure, in all sectors where health workers work;
- Implement a surveillance and prevention programme for accidental exposure to mbpc;
- Carry out continuous surveillance, encouraging the reporting of accidents;
- Carry out a survey of accidents, risk factors, categories of professionals involved in accidents, and the sectors where accidents occur most frequently, in order to guide the measures to be taken to prevent and control accidents;
- Carrying out training for professionals new to the service, as well as retraining for others;
- Adopt, after careful risk/cost/benefit assessment, safety devices such as needles and syringes with safety locks/caps or retractable mechanisms, needleless systems, safe catheters for peripheral puncture, blind needles for suturing as required by NR32;
- Supply and replace PPE in quantity and quality for use by its professionals;
- Provide a sufficient quantity and quality of containers for the disposal of sharps and mbpc;
- Properly manage solid and liquid healthcare waste;
- Define a protocol with the procedures to be adopted in the event of accidental exposure to mbpc;
- Provide written guidance to healthcare professionals on the

procedures to be adopted in the event of accidental exposure to mbpc;
- Post a protocol with the procedures to be adopted in the event of accidental exposure to

mbpc in visible and strategic locations;

- Require a vaccination card when hiring a professional to work in the health area that involves direct contact with patients and indirect contact with blood and its derivatives, body fluids, secretions and excretions and mbpc. If the professional does not present a document recording their full immunisation schedule, they must request that their vaccinations be updated before starting work. The service itself must track this process.

c) Government

In Brazil, there are two latest instruments for protecting workers: Ordinance No. 777 of 2004 from the Ministry of Health and NR 32 of 2005 from the Ministry of Labour and Employment.

Ordinance 777/2004 provides for compulsory notification of various occupational health problems to a specific sentinel service network, including accidents involving biological material; it stipulates that notification should be made via SINAN and that the Sentinel Network for Compulsory Notification of Work-Related Accidents and Diseases should be created, with the aim of integrating assistance and surveillance actions for occupational health (BRASIL, 2004).

The purpose of Regulatory Standard NR32 is to establish the basic guidelines for implementing measures to protect the health and safety of health service workers, as well as those who carry out health promotion and care activities in general. Among other guidelines, this standard emphasises biological risk, in its Annex II, ongoing training for workers and mandatory vaccination against tetanus, diphtheria and hepatitis B.

Other important items include personal hygiene principles, signposting, labelling, personal and collective protective equipment and emergency procedures, which will ensure greater safety for workers (BRASIL, 2005b). Among these items, we need to highlight the mandatory use of intravenous catheters with safety devices and needle-free systems, which is essential to make the procedure and the environment safer.

Ordinances and resolutions are important instruments that establish basic obligations and guidelines for various actions, but their incorporation into everyday life is often lacking.

You have to realise that these instruments were created to protect the workers themselves. It's a legal instrument to protect workers. It's important to follow them.

CHAPTER 6

CONCLUSION

The first stage of the study sought to identify accidental exposure to occupational hazards among professionals in the mobile APH health team working on highways, in which 4,992 roadside assistance forms (FAR) were analysed. Fifty-four exposures to occupational risks were detected, of which only six (11.1%) were notified to the SEESMT. Among the accidental exposures to occupational risks among the professionals in the mobile APH team, the risk of an accident stood out (64.8%), followed by non-ergonomic situations (16.7%) and biological risks (9.2%). Physical and chemical risks occurred less frequently. The most frequent types of accidents faced by mobile APH professionals, in terms of the risk of accidents, were: car collisions (28.6%), aggression from the victim, family members and users (14.3%) and falls, slips during access/approach to the victim (11.4%).

In the second stage, which analysed accidental exposure to potentially contaminated biological material (pbm) in mobile APH healthcare team professionals, it was found that of the 50 mobile APH team professionals interviewed, 28 (56%) reported accidental exposure to some type of potentially contaminated biological material, making a total of 41 accidents.

As for the characterisation of the mobile APH professionals taking part in the study, the majority (38%) were aged between 20 and 30 years old; males predominated (84%). With regard to professional category, there was a predominance of firefighters (30%), followed by nursing technicians (24%); professional training time of 120 months or more (46%) or more; the majority (56%) had worked in mobile APH for between six (6) and 60 months; (80%) worked in mobile APH on motorways; and the majority (92%) had a full HBV vaccination programme.

The professional category most exposed to mbpc accidents was doctors (83.3 per cent), followed by nurses (75 per cent), firefighters (66.7 per cent), nursing technicians (41.7 per cent), and finally drivers (22.2 per cent).

Of the accidents, the majority (70.7%) affected intact skin, followed by percutaneous (17.1%); mucous membranes (7.3%) and damaged skin (4.9%).

The majority of accidents involving mbpc occurred during mobile APH on motorways (90.2%).

The most frequently affected body areas were the forearm (41.4%), followed by the arm (21.9%), hand (21.9%) and face (12.2%). At the time of the accidental exposure, among the most frequent were: patient immobilisation procedure (18); physical examination (12); post-insertion of the needle into the patient (07); tracheal intubation procedure (06); and extrication procedure (06).

Among the situations that favoured accidental exposure in mobile APH, the most cited were: emergency (46.4%); patient agitation (28.6%), rescue operation (25%), distraction (21.4%) and stress (17.9%).

Almost all of the professionals said they were wearing denim overalls (95.1%) or specific fire approach clothing and a helmet (4.1%) and long boots (90.2%) when the accident occurred. The majority reported wearing latex/procedure gloves (63.4%). The other most commonly used PPE was goggles (24.4%) and a face mask (14.6%).

As for the immediate action taken at the site exposed to the mbpc, the majority (43.9%) washed with soap and water, followed by the use of antiseptic (41.5%), water alone (7.3%), and no action at all (7.3%).

Of the 41 exposures to mbpc, 12 (29.3%) professionals sought medical advice; seven (25%) underwent serological tests for HCV, HBV and HIV; one required prophylaxis for HIV and another for HCV; and 70.7% did not take any action because they believed there was no need. Of these accidents, the majority (78.1%) did not report the accident at work (CAT).

With regard to the existence of rules for the prevention and control of accidents with biological material and the protocol for behaviour after accidental exposure to mbpc in the service, almost all of them were positive, i.e. 94% and 96% respectively; 96% said they had received training on occupational risks in mobile APH and PPE.

All (100 per cent) of the professionals reported that ambulances are cleaned with soap and water; (98 per cent) reported using sodium hypochlorite.

As for how they disinfected the material, 96% reported soap and water, 96% sodium hypochlorite and 4.0% glutaraldehyde.

With regard to the form of packaging used for sharps, the majority (88 per cent) reported disposing of them in appropriate cardboard rubbish bins with rigid, impermeable walls.

According to the mobile APH professionals, 98 per cent reported disposing of solid waste in hospital rubbish and liquid waste in the sewer (54 per cent).

As for the factors that favour the occurrence of accidental exposure to biological risks in mobile APH, several were mentioned by the professionals on the mobile APH team, involving those related to the location of the accident, user care, physical space, environment, experience in the field, and biopsycho-emotional factors, among them: vehicle flow, agitated victims, places that are difficult to access, lack of training in mobile APH, stress, among others.

Several suggestions were made by professionals from the mobile APH team, which partly subsidised the suggestions for strategies to prevent and control accidental exposure to mbpc, outlined as part of the contribution of this study.

The results show the vulnerability of mobile APH team professionals to occupational risks in general. Analysing the results relating to mbpc accidents, the main focus of this study, highlighted some of the various problems surrounding this issue. There is still much to explore, as studies of this nature are still in their infancy. This study only shows results obtained in one company. It is necessary for each service, company and institution to carry out its own self-assessment to find out the extent of the problem, the activities at risk, diagnose its needs and establish an action plan, based on its data, with the aim of promoting safety for its workers, minimising the risks of accidental exposure to mbpc and providing adequate care for mobile APH professionals exposed to accidents.

CHAPTER 7

REFERENCES

ABREU, A.M.M.; MAURO, M.Y.C. Accidents at work among nursing staff in the emergency department of a municipal hospital in Rio de Janeiro. Esc. Anna Nery R. Enferm. Rio de Janeiro, v. 4, n.1, p. 139-146, Apr. 2000.

AGUIAR, K. N.; SILVA, A. L. A. C.; FARIA, C. R.; LIMA, F. V.; SOUZA, P. R.; STACCIARINI, J. M. R. - Stress in a military pre-hospital rescue team. Rev. Eletrônica de Enfermagem, Goiânia, v. 2, n.2, jul./dez. 2000. Available at: <http://www.revistas.ufg.br/index.php/fen.> Accessed on: 22 September 2008.

ALVES, D. W.; BISSEL, R.A. Bacterial pathogens in ambulance: results of unannounced sample collection. Prehospital emergency care, v.12, n. 2, p. 218-224, 2008.

ANDRADE, D.; ANGERANI, E.L.S.; PADOVANI, C.R. Microbiological conditions of hospital beds before and after cleaning. Rev. Saúde Publ. v. 34, n. 2, p.163-169, Apr. 2000.

BRAZILIAN ASSOCIATION OF TECHNICAL STANDARDS - ABNT. NBR 15292: Made-up articles, high-visibility safety clothing. Rio de Janeiro, 2005.

BRAZILIAN ASSOCIATION OF TECHNICAL STANDARDS - ABNT. NBR 14561: vehicles for emergency medical care and rescue. Rio de Janeiro, 2000. Available at: <http://www.abnt.org.br/cb24/relacao_normas.html>. Accessed on: 09 June 2008.

ASSOCIAÇÃO PAULISTA DE ESTUDOS E CONTROLE DE INFECÇÃO HOSPITALAR - APECIH. Guidelines for infection control in healthcare personnel. São Paulo: APECIH, 1998.

BACHION et al. Stress, anxiety and coping: a review of concepts, measures and intervention strategies for nursing practice. REME. Revista Mineira de Enfermagem, Belo Horizonte, v. 2, n. 1, p. 33-39, 1998.

BALDY, J.L.S. Immunisation of health professionals and hospitalised patients. In: RODRIGUES, E.A.C. et al. Infecções hospitalares: prevenção e controle. São Paulo: Sarvier, 1997. p. 367-372.

BALSAMO, A.C. Study on accidents at work involving exposure to human body fluids in health workers. 2002. 137f. Dissertation (Master's) - School of Nursing, University of São Paulo, São Paulo, 2002.

BALSAMO, A.C; BARRIENTOS, D.S.; ROSSI, J.C.B. Accidents at work involving exposure to human bodily fluids among employees of the University Hospital of São Paulo (HU - USP). Revista de Medicina do HU-USP, São Paulo, v. 10, n.1, p. 39-45, jan./jun., 2000.

BALSAMO, A.C. FELLI, V.E.A. Estudo sobre os acidentes de trabalho com exposição aos líquidos corporais humanos em trabalhadores de saúde de um hospital universitário. Rev. latino-am. enfermagem, Ribeirão Preto, v. 14, n. 3, 2006. Available at: <http://www.scielosp.org/scielo>. Accessed on: 18 Nov. 2007.

BARBOZA, D.B.; SOLER, Z.A.S.G.; CIORLIA, L.A.S. Work accidents with sharps involving the nursing staff of a teaching hospital. Arquivos de Ciências da Saúde, São José do Rio Preto, v. 11, n. 2, p. 2-8, Apr./Jun., 2004.

BASSO, M. Occupational accidents involving blood and other bodily fluids in health professionals. 1999. 112f. Dissertation (Master's) - Ribeirão Preto School of Nursing, University of São Paulo, Ribeirão Preto, 1999.

BENATTI, M.C.C. Accidents at work among nursing workers in a university hospital. Rev. Esc. Enferm. USP, São Paulo, v. 35, n. 2, p. 155-162, jun. 2001.

BIOSECURITY: there's no such thing as too little care. REVISTA EMERGENCIA. p.56-61, March 2007.

BRAGA, D. Accidente de trabalho com material biológico em trabalhadores da equipe de enfermagem do Centro de Pesquisas Hospital Evandro Chagas. 2000, 75f. Dissertation (Master's Degree) - Oswaldo Cruz Foundation, National School of Public Health, Rio de Janeiro, 2000.

BRANDI, S.S; BENATTI, M.C.C; ALEXANDRE, N.M.C. Occurrence of accidents at work involving sharps among nursing workers in a hospital in the city of Campinas, state of São Paulo. Rev. Esc. Enferm. USP. São Paulo, v.32, n.2, p. 124-33, 1998.

BRAZIL. Federal Council of Medicine. The inter-hospital transport of patients and other measures: 1596/2000. Diário Oficial da União; Poder Executivo, Brasília, DF, n. 116, 16 June 2000. Section, p. 68. Available at: http://www.cremesp.org.br. Accessed on: 23 June 2008.

BRAZIL. Federal Council of Medicine. Establishes structures for providing urgent and emergency care in public and private emergency rooms: 1451/1995. Diário Oficial da União; Poder Executivo, Brasília, DF, n. 17 mar., 1995. Section 1, p. 3666. Available at: http://www.cremesp.org.br. Accessed on: 22 Nov 2008.

_____. Ministry of Health. Ordinance no. 2048 of 5 November 2002. The technical regulation of state urgency and emergency systems. Official Gazette of the Federative Republic of Brazil, Executive Branch, Brasília, DF, 12 November 2002. Section I, p. 3254. Available at: <http://elegis.bvs.br/leisref/public/showAct.php?id=19024&word=abstinencia#'>. Accessed on: 6 May 2006.

_____. Ministry of Health. Ordinance no. 777 of 28 April 2004. Technical procedures for compulsory notification of occupational health problems in a specific sentinel service network, in the Unified Health System - SUS Available at:< http://www.saude.df.gov.br/sites/100/163/00004320.doc>. Accessed on: 27 May 2008.

. Ministry of Health. Social Communications Office. Five-year health plan 1990/95: the health of the new Brazil. Brasília: Ministry of Health Documentation Centre, 1991. 79p.

_____. Ministry of Health. Hospital Infection Control Coordination.
Processing of articles and surfaces in health establishments. 2. ed. Brasília: Ministério da Saúde, 1994a. 49p.

_____. Ministry of Health. Recommendations for care and follow-up of occupational exposure to biological material: HIV and hepatitis B and C. Brasília, DF, 2004b. 56p. Available at:<http://www.aids.gov.br/final/biblioteca/manual_exposicao/manual_acidentes.doc> Accessed on: 27 May 2006.

_____. Ministry of Health. Secretariat for Health Policies. National STD and AIDS Coordination. Manual of behaviour: occupational exposure to biological material: hepatitis and HIV. Brasília, 20p., 1999.

_____. Ministry of Health. Secretariat for Health Policies. National STD and AIDS Coordination. Recommendations for antiretroviral therapy in HIV-infected adults and adolescents. Brasília, 2005a.

_____. Ministry of Labour and Employment. Ordinance no. 485 of 11 November 2005. NR 32- Safety and health at work in health services Brazil, 2005b. Available at: <http://www.mte.gov.br>. Accessed on: 11 May 2007.

_____. Ministry of Health. Processing of articles and surfaces in health establishments. 2. ed. Brasília: MEC, 1994b. 50p.

_____. Ministry of Health. Health Care Secretariat. Department of Strategic Programme Actions. Exposure to biological materials. Brasília: Ministry of Health Publishing House, 76p. 2006. Available at: <http: //www.saude.gov.br/trabalhador>. Accessed on: 03 de 25 nov. 2008.

BREVIDELLI, M.M; CIANCIARULLO, T.I. Analysis of needlestick accidents in a university hospital: occurrence situations and trends. Rev. latino-am. enfermagem. Ribeirão Preto, v. 10, n. 6, p. 780-6, nov./dez., 2002.
BULHÕES, I. Riscos do trabalho de enfermagem. 2. ed. Rio de Janeiro: Folha Carioca, 1998. 278p.

CAIXETA, R. de B.; BARBOSA-BRANCO, A. Occupational accidents involving biological material among health professionals in public hospitals in the Federal District. Cad. Saúde Públ , Rio de Janeiro, v. 21, n.3, p.737- 46, maio/jun., 2005.

CANALLI, R.T.C. Accidents involving biological material among nursing students in a municipality in the interior of São Paulo. 2008. 124f. Dissertation (Master's) - Ribeirão Preto School of Nursing, University of São Paulo, Ribeirão Preto, 2008.

CANINI, S.R.M.S. et al. Sharps accidents among nursing workers at a university hospital in the interior of São Paulo. Rev. latino-am. enfermagem. Ribeirão Preto, v. 10, n. 2, p. 172-8, mar./abr., 2002.

CENTRES FOR DISEASE CONTROL AND PREVENTION (CDC). Transmission of hepatitis B and C viruses in outpatient settings, New York, Oklahoma, and Nebraska, 20002002. MMWR, Atlanta, v. 52, n. 38, p. 901-923, Sep. 2003. Available at: <http://www.cdc.gov./mmwr/preview/mm>. Accessed on: 21 May 2006.

_______. Universal precautions for prevention of transmission of human immunodeficiency virus, hepatitis B virus, and other blood borne pathogens in health-care-settings. MMWR, v.37, n. 24, p. 377-88, 1988.

_______. Updated U.S. public health service guidelines for the management of occupational exposure to HBV, HCV, and HIV and recommendations for postexposure prophylaxis. MMWR, Atlanta, v. 50, n. RR11, p.1-42, jun. 2001. Available at: <http://www.cdc.gov/mmwr/preview/mmwrhtml>. Accessed on: 5 May 2006.

_______. Update: provisional public health services recommendat ions for chemoprophylaxis after occupational exposure to HIV. MMWR, v. 45, n. 45, p. 46872, 1996.

_______. Recommendations for prevention of HIV transmission in the health-care settings. MMWR, v. 36, n. 2, p. 3-17, 1987.

_______. Guidelines for Isolation Precautions: preventing transmission of infectious agents in health-care settings, 2007. Updated in June 2007. Available at: http://www.cdc.gov. Accessed on: 23 September 2008.

CIORLIA, L.A.S.; ZANETTA, D.M.T. Hepatitis C in health professionals: prevalence and association with risk factors. Rev. Saúde Publ. v. 41, n. 2, p. 229-235, 2007.

COSTA M.A.F; COSTA M.F.B. Biosafety from A to Z. Rio de Janeiro: Papel virtual; 2003.186p.

DESLANDES, S.F. et al. Conceptions of risk and prevention from the perspective of injecting drug users. Cad. Saúde Públ. Rio de Janeiro, v.18, n.1, p. 141-151, jan/feb. 2002.

FERNANDES, R.J. Characterisation of mobile pre-hospital care in the health department of the municipality of Ribeirão Preto-SP. 2004. 101f. Dissertation (Master's) - Ribeirão Preto School of Nursing, University of São Paulo, Ribeirão Preto, 2004.

FERREIRA, A.B.H. Novo Aurélio: o dicionário da língua portuguesa do século XX. 3. ed. Rio de Janeiro: Nova Fronteira, 1999a. p. 302.

FERREIRA, C.S.W. Emergency care services in the Municipality of São Paulo: implementation of a pre-hospital care system. São Paulo, 1999b, 110f.
Dissertation (Master's Degree) - Department of Preventive Medicine, Faculty of Medicine, University of São Paulo, São Paulo, 1999b.

FIGUEIREDO, J. Emergência: condutas médicas e transportes. Rio de Janeiro: Guanabara Koogan, 1996. p. 36-48.

FLORÊNCIO, V.B.; RODRIGUES, C.; PEREIRA, M.S.; SOUZA, A.C.S. Adherence to standard precautions among professionals in the pre-hospital rescue team of the Goiás Fire Department. Rev. Eletrônica de Enfermagem, v. 5 n. 1, p. 43-8, 2003. Available at: < http://www.revistas.ufg.br/index.php/fen> Accessed on: 10 Aug. 2008.

GARNER, J.S. Guideline for isolation precautions in hospitals. Infect. Control. Hosp. Epidemiol. v.1, n.17, p. 54-80, 1996.

GALAFASSI, M.C. Medicina do trabalho: programa de controle médico de saúde ocupacional (NR-7). 2. ed. São Paulo: Atlas, 1999. 164 p.

GALIZZI FILHO, J. Current aspects of the diagnosis and treatment of chronic hepatitis B in monoinfected patients. Jornal Brasileiro de AIDS, São Paulo, v. 8, n.1, p. 23-33, jan./feb., 2007.

GERBERDING, J. L. Occupational exposure to HIV in health care settings. N. Engl. J. Med. v. 348, n. 9, p. 826-833, 2003. Available at: <http://www.nejm.org>. Accessed on: 4 June 2006.

GERBERDING, J.L. Management of occupational exposures to blood-borne viruses. The New England Journal of Medicine.v. 332, n.7, p. 444 - 451, feb. 1995.

GIR, E.; COSTA, F.P.P.; SILVA, A.M.A. A enfermagem frente a acidentes de trabalho com material potencialmente contaminado na era do HIV. Rev. Esc. Enferm USP. São Paulo, v. 32, n.3, p. 262-272, oct. 1998.

HISTORY OF THE AMBULANCE. RI Rev Intensiva. n. 4, p. 107, feb./abr., 2006.

HOEFEL, H.H.K. Ambulance and infection control. n.d. Available at: <http://www.cih.com.br/transporte>. Accessed on: 18 May 2006.

KITAYAMA, C.V.; MARÍNGOLO, E.F. Accidents with potentially infected material: nursing students' perception of vulnerability. Ribeirão Preto, 2000. 83f. Course Conclusion Paper (Bachelor's Degree in Nursing). Nursing Course, Barão de Mauá University Centre, Ribeirão Preto, 2000.

LOPES, A.C.S. et al. Adherence to standard precautions by mobile pre-hospital care staff in Belo Horizonte, MG, Brazil. Cad. Saúde Pública, Rio de Janeiro, v. 24, n. 6, p. 1387-96. 2008.

LOPES, L.K.O. et al. Care for professional victims of accidents with biological material in an infectious diseases hospital. Rev. Eletrônica de Enfermagem, v.6, n.3, 2004. Available at: <http://www.fen.ufg.br>. Accessed on: 20 May 2006.

MACHADO, A.A. Factors related to adherence in healthcare workers who have suffered an occupational accident involving biological risk. 2006. Ribeirão Preto, 2006, 162f. Thesis (Livre docência). Ribeirão Preto Medical School, University of São Paulo, Ribeirão Preto, 2006.

MAFRA et al. Nurses' perception of the importance of using personal protective equipment for biological risks in a mobile emergency care service.
O mundo da saúde São Paulo, v.32, n. 1, p. 31-38, 2008.

MANETTI, M.T.; COSTA, J.C.S.; MARZIALE, M.H.P.; TROVÓ, M.E. Presence of accidents at work involving biological material according to the Green and Kreuter model. Rev. Gaúcha Enferm, Porto Alegre - RS, v. 27, n. 1, p. 80-91, 2006.

MARZIALE, M.H.P. Underreporting of sharps accidents in nursing. Rev. Bras. Enferm., Brasília, v. 56, n. 2, p. 164-8, mar./abr., 2003.

MARZIALE, M.H.P., NISHIMURA, K.Y.N., FERREIRA, M.M. Risks of contamination caused by accidents at work with sharps among nursing workers. Rev. latino-am. enfermagem, São Paulo, v.12, n.1, p. 36-42, 2004. Available at: <http://www.scielo.br/pdf/rlae>. Accessed on: 7 June 2006.

MENDES, R. Pathologia do trabalho. 2ª ed. São Paulo: Atheneu, 2003. p.1443-500.

MOREIRA, C.O.F. Between the individual and society: a study of John Dewey's philosophy of education. Bragança Paulista: EDUSF, 2002. 217p.

MOYA, A.C. Sanitary evacuation under conditions of biosafety. Emergencies, n.19, p. 144-150, 2007

MUROFUSE, N.T.; MARZIALE, M.H.P.; GEMELLI, L.M.G. Accident with biological material in a university hospital in western Paraná. Rev. Gaúcha Enferm, Porto Alegre - RS, v. 26, n. 2, p. 168-79, 2005.

NAPOLEÃO, A.A. Causes of underreporting of accidents at work: the view of nursing workers at a hospital in the interior of São Paulo. 1999. 115f. Dissertation (Master's) - Ribeirão Preto School of Nursing, University of São Paulo, Ribeirão Preto, 1999.

NETTINA, S.M. Brunner. Nursing practice. 7. ed. Rio de Janeiro: Guanabara Koogan, v. 2, 2003.

NHAMBA, L.A. Occupational accidents with biological material among nursing professionals in a hospital in Angola. 2004. 117f. Dissertation (Master's) - Ribeirão Preto School of Nursing, University of São Paulo, Ribeirão Preto, 2004.

NICHIATA et al. Evolution of isolation in communicable diseases: knowledge in contemporary practice. Rev. Enferm. USP. v. 38, n.1, p.61-70, 2004.

NISHIDE, V.M.; BENATTI, M.C.C. Occupational risks among nursing workers in an Intensive Care Unit. Rev. Esc. Enferm. USP. v. 38, n. 4, 406-414, 2004.

NITSCHKE, C.A.S.; LOPES, N.G.; BUENO, R.M.L. Labour risks in a mobile Intensive Care Unit. 2000. 81f. Monograph (Specialisation) - Federal University of Santa Catarina, Santa Catarina, 2000.

OLIVEIRA, F.A. et al. Human accidents caused by Africanised bee stings. Rev. Soc. Bras. Med. Trop. Uberaba, v. 33, n. 4, 2000. Available at: <http://www.scielo.br/scielo. Accessed on: 25 October 2008.

WORLD HEALTH ORGANISATION-WHO. Framework to reduce the burden of TB/HIV. Translation by Paula Perdigão. Genoa, 2002.

PAN-AMERICAN HEALTH ORGANISATION. Chemical accidents: Health aspects. Guide to preparedness and response. Pan American Health Organisation. Washington, D.C., 1998.

OLIVEIRA, N.B.; SOUZA, R.M.C. Diagnosis of injuries and quality of life of motorcyclists, victims of traffic accidents. Rev. latino-am. enfermagem, Ribeirão Preto, v.11, n. 6, p.750, nov/dez., 2003.

PATRICK, R. Ouch! Sharps and the needle-stick challenge. Emergency medical Services, v. 33, n.10, p. 139, 2004.

PEREIRA, M.S.; MORIYA, T.M. Infecção hospitalar: estrutura básica de vigilância e controle. 2.ed.Goiânia: AB, 1994. 193p.

PREVENTION OF ACCIDENTS WITH VENOMOUS ANIMALS. Butantã Institute. São Paulo, 2001. Available at: <http://www.butantan.gov.br/pop/prevencao_acidentes.pdf> Accessed on: 25 October 2008.

PRISTA J; UVA. A.S. Occupational exposure to chemical agents: biological indicators in workers' health surveillance. Rev. portuguesa de saúde pública, v. 18, n.1. p. 59, jan./jun., 2000. Available at: http://www.ensp.unl.pt/ensp/corpo- docente/websites_docentes/sousa_uva/sousa_uva. Accessed on: 8 October 2008.

RAPPARINI, C.; CARDO, D.M. Main infectious diseases diagnosed in health professionals. In: MASTROIENI, M.F. Biosafety applied to laboratories and health services. São Paulo: Atheneu, 2004. chap. 2, p. 205-18.

REIS, J.N.; CORREA, A.K. Emergency unit: stress x communication. In: Brazilian Symposium on Nursing Communication, 2. 1990. Ribeirão Preto. Proceedings... Ribeirão Preto: Ribeirão Preto School of Nursing. University of São Paulo, 1990. 528-38

REIS, R.K.; GIR, E.; CANINI, S.R.M.S. Accidents with biological material among undergraduate nursing students in a public Brazilian university. Brasilian Journal of Infectious Diseases, Salvador, v. 8, n. 1, p. 18-24, feb. 2004.

RESENDE, M.R. Tuberculosis: risk in health professionals, 2004. Available at: <http://www.riscobiologico.org/patogenos/tb.asp>. Accessed on: 22 April 2007.

RIBEIRO FILHO, N. Management of Health Service Waste. In: Fernandes, A.T.; Fernandes.M.O.V.; Ribeiro F. N. Infecção Hospitalar e suas Interfaces na Área de Saúde. São Paulo (SP): Atheneu, 2000, p.1156-1200.

RIBEIRO, P.H.V. Accidents with potentially contaminated biological material in students of a dentistry course in the interior of the state of Paraná. Ribeirão Preto, 2005. 150f. Master's dissertation. Faculty of Health Sciences, University of São Paulo, Ribeirão Preto, 2005.

ROBAZZI, M.L.C.C.; SILVEIRA, C.A.; MARZIALE, M.H.P. Hospital records helping to identify violence at work. Rev. Enferm. UERJ. v. 14, n.4, p. 409505, 2006.

RODRIGUES, A.B.; MAGALHÃES, M.B.B.; SALES, S.M.M. The issue of the human immunodeficiency virus and self-protection at work. Rev. bras. Enferm. v. 48, n. 3, p.272-285, jul./set., 1995.

ROUQUAYROL, M. Z.; ALMEIDA FILHO, N. Epidemiologia & Saude. 5ª . ed. Rio de Janeiro: MEDSI, 1999. 570p.

RUIZ, M.T.; BARBOZA, D.B.; SOLER, Z.Z.G. Accidentes de trabalho: um estudo sobre esta ocorrência em hospital geral. Arquivos de Ciências da Saúde, São José do Rio Preto, v. 11, n. 4, p. 219-224, Oct./Dec., 2004.

SAILER, G.C. Adesão de trabalhadores de enfermagem ao tratamento com os anti- retrovirais pós-exposição ocupacional a material biológico. 2004. 130f. Dissertation (Master's) - Ribeirão Preto School of Nursing, University of São Paulo, Ribeirão Preto, 2004. Available at: <http://www.teses.usp.br/teses>. Accessed on: 9 May 2006.

SANTOS, E.M. dos; ARAÚJO, T.M. de. Work process and workers' health at the Professor Edgard Santos University Hospital - HUPES. Revista Baiana de Saúde Pública, Salvador, v. 27, n. 2, p. 143-154, jul./dez., 2003.

SANTOS, I.F. Biological risks: analysis and proposals for prevention at the Hospital das Clínicas de Marília - SP. 2002. 156f Thesis (Doctorate) - Ribeirão Preto Nursing School, University of São Paulo, Ribeirão Preto, 2002.

SANTOS, B.V.G; SANTOS, A.D. Perfil dos acidentes de trabalho com material de risco biológico envolvendo trabalhadores da área de saúde que atuam no Hospital Universitário Professor Alberto Antunes/UFAL, 58., 2006. Florianópolis. Proceedings... Florianópolis: Auditorium of the Professor Alberto Antunes University Hospital, 2006.

SANTOS, N.J.S.; MONTEIRO, A.L.; RUIZ, E.A.C. The first case of due to occupational in Brazil. Brazilian Journal of Infectious Diseases, v.6, n.3, p. 140-1, jun., 2002.

São Paulo State Government. Transport Regulatory Agency of State of São Paulo - ARTESP. Concessions and permits (1998). Available at: <http://www.artesp.sp.gov.br>. Accessed on: 15 October 2006.

______. Government of the State of São Paulo. Secretariat of Public Management. Provision of hospital cleaning services. v.7, n. 2, p.117, Apr., 2008. Available at: <http://www.cadterc.sp.gov.br>. Accessed on: 26 May 2008.

______. State Department of Health. STD/AIDS Programme. Biological accidents: changes in surveillance, care and prevention. Epidemiological Bulletin, year I, n. 1, January 2007.

SARQUIS, L.M.M.; FELLI, V.E.A. O uso dos equipamentos de proteção individual entre os trabalhadores de enfermagem acidentados com instrumentos perfurocortantes. Rev. Bras. de Enferm, v. 53, n. 4, p. 564-73, dec. 2000.

SCOTTI, C.T.; AGUILERA, M.G.; SILVA, V.A. Accident with biological material: risk factors involved and post-exposure behaviours among nursing students. Ribeirão Preto, 2002. 37f. Course Conclusion Paper (Bachelor's Degree in Nursing). Nursing Course, Barão de Mauá University Centre, Ribeirão Preto, 2002.

SÊCCO, I.A.O. et al. Accidents at work and occupational risks in the day-to-day life of hospital workers: a challenge for workers' health. Espaço para Saúde, Londrina. v. 4, n. 1, 2005. Available at: <http://www.ccs.uel.br>. Accessed on: 11 May 2007.

SEIDEL et al. MOSBY: Guide to physical examination. In:.6. Ed. Rio de Janeiro: Elsevier, 2007. 1040p.

SECRETARIAT OF THE ENVIRONMENT, 2008. Available at: http://www.cetesb.sp.gov/emergencia/aspectos/aspectos_toxologia.asp Accessed on 30 September 2008.

SILVA, M.F.I. Health service waste: management in the operating theatre, materials centre and anaesthetic recovery centre of a hospital in the interior of São Paulo.
2004. 107f. Thesis (Doctorate) - Ribeirão Preto School of Nursing, University of São Paulo, Ribeirão Preto, 2004. Available at: <http://www.teses.usp.br/teses>. Accessed on: 15 Nov. 2008.

SKOVGAARD, P. The journal of infection control nursing. Ambulance watch. Nurs. Times, v. 85, n.49, p. 63-67, dec., 1989. Available at: <http://www.pubmed.com.br/pubmed.php. > Accessed on:

08 May 2007.

SOERENSEN, A.A.; MORIYA, T.M; ROBAZZI, M.L.C.C.; SOERENSEN, R. Mobile pre-hospital care: occupational risk factors. Rev. enferm. UERJ, Apr. 2008, vol.16, n. 2, p.187-192.

SOSNIN, M.; YOUNG, D.; DUNT, D.R. A study of emergency ambulance utilisation. Austr. Fam. Phys. v.18, n.3, p. 233-238, Mar., 1989.

SOUZA, A.C.S. Biological risk and biosafety in the daily lives of nurses and nursing assistants. 2001. 184f. Thesis (Doctorate) - Ribeirão Preto School of Nursing, University of São Paulo, Ribeirão Preto, 2001. Available at: <http://www.teses.usp.br/teses>. Accessed on: 20 Nov. 2008

SOUZA, M. de; VIANA, L. do A.C. Occupational accidents in the nursing team: a study in five hospitals in the municipality of São Paulo. Acta Paulista Enfermagem, São Paulo, v. 13, special issue, part II, p. 58-61, 2000.

SPEERS, D. Infection diseases and the pre-hospital practitioner. Journal of emergency primary health care, v.1, n.1-2,2003.

TAKAYANAGUI, A.M.M.; MENDES, M.M.; DIAS, L. Biosafety, nursing and health service waste. Revista Brasileira de Saúde Ocupacional, São Paulo, v. 21, n. 80, p. 23-27, Oct./Dec., 1993.

TAKEDA, E. Occupational risks, accidents at work and morbidity among drivers at an ambulance centre in the state of São Paulo. 2002. 186f. Dissertation (Master's) - Ribeirão Preto School of Nursing, University of São Paulo, Ribeirão Preto, 2002.

TAKEDA, E.; ROBAZZI, M.L.C.C. Accidents at work among ambulance drivers who provide emergency assistance. Rev. latino-am. enfermagem. Enferm. v. 15, n.3, p. 439445, May/June 2007.

TARANTOLA, A.; ABITEBOUL, D.; RACHLINE, A. Infection risks following accidental exposure to blood or body fluids in health care workers: a review of pathogens transmitted in published cases. Am. J Infect Control. v.34, n.6, p.367-75, 2006.

TEIXEIRA, P; VALLE, S. Biosafety: a multidisciplinary approach. In: ODA, L.M; ROCHA, S.S. da; TEIXIERA, P. AIDS as an occupational disease. Rio de Janeiro: FIOCRUZ, 1996, p. 239-256.

TENGAN, F.M. Risk factors associated with hepatitis C virus infection.1997. 139f. Thesis (Doctorate) - Faculty of Medicine, University of São Paulo, São Paulo, 1997.

TOMAZIN, C.C. et al. Accidents at work involving sharps in nursing workers. Revista Gaúcha de Enfermagem, Porto Alegre, v. 22, n. 2, p. 60-73, jul., 2001.

VIANA, D.R.S.; LOPES, G.T. Biological risk in pre-hospital care. In: Brazilian Nursing Congress, 57. 2005. Goiânia. Proceedings... Goiânia: Goiânia Convention and Culture Centre, 2005. Available at:
<http://bvsms.saude.gov.br/bvs/publicacoes/57cbe/resumos/739>. Accessed on: 08 May 2007.

WHITAKER, I. Y. Severity of trauma assessed in the pre-hospital phase - analysis of victims of external causes attended by SAMU - RESGATE - SP, 1991. 1993. 78f.
Dissertation (Master's Degree) - Paulista School of Medicine, Federal University of São Paulo, São Paulo, 1993.

WHITAKER, I.Y.; GUTIERREZ, M.G.R. de; KOIZUMI, M.S. Trauma severity assessed in the pre-hospital phase. Rev. Assoc. Med. Bras., São Paulo, v. 44, n. 2, p. 111-119, jun., 1998. Available at: <http://www.scielo.br/scielo.php>. Accessed on: 02 September 2006.

XELEGATI, R.; ROBAZZI, M.L.C.C. Chemical risks to which nursing workers are subjected: a literature review. Rev. latino-am. enfermagem, Ribeirao Preto, v. 11, n.3, p. 350-356, 2003.

YANES et al, Reconverson industrial y salud de los trabajadores. Salud trabajadores, Maracay v.1, n. 1, 6-14, mai., 1993.

ZAPPAROLI, A.; MARZIALE, M. Occupational risk in emergency basic and advanced life support units. Rev Bras Enfermagem. feb./mar. v. 59, n.1 p. 41-6., 2006.

ZOBOLI, E.L.C.P. Bioethics and labour nursing. In: CARVALHO, G.M. et al. Enfermagem do trabalho. São Paulo: EPU, 2001. chap. 7, p. 79-95.

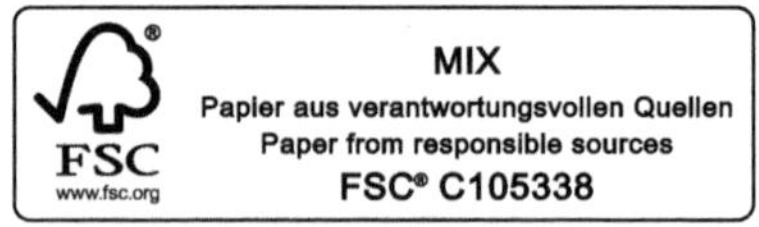

Printed by Books on Demand GmbH, Norderstedt / Germany